D1479553

EUROPEAN SCHOOL OF ONCOLOGY SCIENTIFIC UPDATES, VOLUME 5

Fatigue and Cancer

EUROPEAN SCHOOL OF ONCOLOGY SCIENTIFIC UPDATES

Series Editors: U. Veronesi and M.S. Aapro

EUROPEAN SCHOOL OF ONCOLOGY SCIENTIFIC UPDATES, VOLUME 5

Fatigue and Cancer

Edited by

Michel Marty
Institut Gustave Roussy
Villejuif, France

Sergio Pecorelli
European Institute of Oncology
Milan, Italy

2001

ELSEVIER

AMSTERDAM - LONDON - NEW YORK - OXFORD - PARIS - SHANNON - TOKYO

ELSEVIER SCIENCE B.V.
Sara Burgerhartstraat 25
P.O. Box 211, 1000 AE Amsterdam, The Netherlands

First edition 2001

Library of Congress Cataloging in Publication Data
A catalog record from the Library of Congress has been applied for.

ISBN: 0 444 50905 4

♾ The paper used in this publication meets the requirements of ANSI/NISO Z39.48-1992 (Permanence of Paper).
Printed in The Netherlands.

The European School of Oncology gratefully acknowledges
sponsorship for the Task Force received from

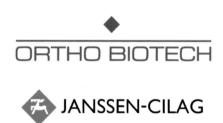

ORTHO BIOTECH

JANSSEN-CILAG

Foreword

The European School of Oncology (ESO) is a non-governmental, non profit-making organisation, which was founded in 1982. It has since become a model for many other professional groups that need to provide timely information, education and training. The rate of progress in the areas of diagnosis and treatment of cancer is so rapid that oncologists need continuous updating in order to provide their patients the best chances for palliation or cure. ESO recognises the multidisciplinary nature of cancer treatment, and its activities encompass all medical, nursing and technical specialities dealing with neoplastic diseases. Timeliness and scientific accuracy are the key factors behind the numerous activities of the School.

One of the many initiatives of ESO has been the institution of study groups, also called task forces, where leading experts exchange views on the state of the art of a given field, discuss controversies and new developments, and give opinions on future directions. These groups often publish a summary in a peer-reviewed journal, or excerpts of the discussions are presented as "Newsletters". The *Scientific Updates* are a series of books designed to disseminate the full results of such discussions. Each issue is under the responsibility of one or several volume editors, and contains the latest information on a particular topic.

To preserve the timeliness of the information, the ESO *Scientific Updates* utilise a simple layout and presentation to enable very rapid publication times, thus overcoming a common problem in the medical literature: that of the material being outdated even before publication.

The editors welcome suggestions for further issues and, together with the whole ESO staff, are ready to help interested parties in establishing new task force meetings. In this way the knowledge of new developments in all fields of oncology, from research through to nursing, can be shared. Education and training are important in helping reduce cancer-related mortality, and the ESO is firmly committed to achieving this aim.

Matti S. Aapro
ESO Scientific Updates
Series Editor

Umberto Veronesi
Chairman Scientific Committee
European School of Oncology

Contents

x

ESO Scientific Updates, Vol. 5
Fatigue and Cancer
M. Marty and S. Pecorelli, editors
© 2001 Elsevier Science B.V. All rights reserved

1

Introduction

Michel Marty and Sergio Pecorelli

Fatigue in cancer patients has only recently emerged as one of the major con-
comitants of cancer and its treatment, perhaps rather surprisingly, as it has a
profound impact on decision making, on health-related quality of life and on
numerous symptom scales. This late recognition may very well be related to the
fact that the mechanisms of fatigue have long been poorly understood and in
the past no specific therapeutic interventions were available.

More recently, fatigue has been better defined, specific grading tools have
been designed and validated, and some knowledge of its complex mechanisms
has been acquired. This has led to the recognition of its incidence in cancer patients and of its impact on their lives, and to the definition of fatigue-oriented
treatment strategies. All these issues are discussed in the present volume.

We cannot yet say that we fully understand and can optimally control fatigue, but we have reached a stage where no oncologist can ignore fatigue in patients with cancer. The clinician should know how to grade fatigue, recognise its
main causes, and be able to design a therapeutic approach, whether it be sub-
tractive, by reducing the causes of fatigue, or additive, by introducing specific
measures to treat it.

These issues formed the basis of a course organised in the autumn of 2000 by
the European School of Oncology (ESO), at which some of the world's experts
shared their experiences, concerns and opinions. Their presentations were collected in the present volume of the ESO Scientific Update series, which we
view as the "vade mecum" on fatigue in cancer patients for oncologists, general
practitioners, and staff involved in cancer patient care.

There is no doubt that this field will undergo rapid evolution and will require periodic updating. This will be incorporated into future ESO courses.

The authors are grateful to ESO for having paved the way for a comprehensive approach to the management of fatigue in cancer patients. This is an important contribution of ESO to the training of oncologists all over the world.

ESO Scientific Updates, Vol. 5
Fatigue and Cancer
M. Marty and S. Pecorelli, editors
© 2001 Elsevier Science B.V. All rights reserved

Impact of Cancer-Related Fatigue on the Lives of Patients: New Findings from the Fatigue Coalition

Gregory A. Curt[1], William Breitbart[2], David Cella[3], Jerome E. Groopman[4], Sandra J. Horning[5], Loretta M. Itri[6], David H. Johnson[7], Christine Miaskowski[8], Susan L. Scherr[9], Russell K. Portenoy[10], and Nicholas J. Vogelzang[11], The Fatigue Coalition

[1]National Cancer Institute, Bethesda, MD; [2]Memorial Sloan-Kettering Cancer Center, New York, NY; [3]Evanston Northwestern Healthcare, Evanston, IL; [4]Harvard Medical School, Beth Israel Deaconess Medical Center, Boston, MA; [5]Stanford University Medical Center, Stanford, CA; [6]Ortho Biotech Inc., Raritan, NJ; [7]Vanderbilt University, Nashville, TN; [8] University of California San Francisco, San Francisco, CA; [9]The National Coalition for Cancer Survivorship, Silver Spring, MD; [10]Beth Israel Medical Center, New York, NY; [11]The University of Chicago, Chicago, IL.

Introduction

Patients with cancer commonly report a lack of energy during the course of their disease and treatment [1]. Fatigue may result from the disease itself, antineoplastic therapies, and/or a broad range of physical and psychologic comorbidities. Fatigue is multidimensional and can be described in terms of perceived energy, mental capacity, and psychologic status [2,3]. It can impair daily functioning and lead to negative effects on quality of life [4-7], self-care capabilities [8], and desire to continue treatment [9]. In some cases, fatigue is the most significant barrier to functional recovery in cancer patients with stable disease who are undergoing chemotherapy [10].

The incidence and severity of cancer-related fatigue appear to be influenced by characteristics of the patient [9,11-13], primary malignancy, and type/intensity of treatment [2]. Fatigue has been reported in 80% to 99% of cancer patients who undergo treatment with chemotherapy, radiotherapy, or both [5,12,14,15]. Although the relative importance of physical (e.g. anemia, cachexia), psycho-

Presented at the thirty-fifth annual meeting of the American Society of Clinical Oncology, Atlanta, GA, May 15-18, 1999

Reproduced with permission from Curt G et al. Impact of Cancer-Related Fatigue on the Lives of Patients: New Findings from the Fatigue Coalition. The Oncologist 2000; 5: 353-60, ©AlphaMed Press 1083-7159

Address for correspondence: G.A. Curt, National Cancer Institute, 12N214 Room Bldg 10, Bethesda, MD 20892-0001, USA. Tel.: +1-301-4964251, fax: +1-301-4969962, e-mail: curtg@mail.nih.gov

logical (e.g. depression, anxiety), and situational (e.g. sleep deprivation) factors usually is unclear [2,9,10,14,16,17], these and other factors appear to be important in the pathogenesis and may be predominant in some cases.

Interest in characterizing the epidemiology and pathogenesis of cancer-related fatigue has intensified in recent years [2]. Research on this subject has been limited, however, and evaluation of data from previous studies is complicated by variations in defining and assessing fatigue and its relatively high prevalence in the general population [10,17]. Recent acceptance of cancer-related fatigue as a diagnosis in the International Classification of Diseases 10th Revision-Clinical Modification (ICD-10) should help ensure a standardized diagnosis in research settings and clinical practice [2,3].

The Fatigue Coalition, a multidisciplinary group of medical practitioners/researchers (oncology, HIV/AIDS, palliative care, psychiatry, psychology) and patient advocates, was formed to study the incidence, prevalence, and functional impact of fatigue in patients with cancer and to develop diagnosis and treatment guidelines (see Appendix). In 1996 we conducted the first large-scale, population-based survey to characterize the epidemiology of cancer-related fatigue and its impact from the perspectives of patients, primary caregivers, and oncologists [6]. Data from that tripart survey confirmed that fatigue is highly prevalent, causes substantial functional and psychological impairment, and is rarely discussed or treated. In an effort to better understand the nature of cancer-related fatigue in patients receiving chemotherapy, we conducted a second survey specifically designed to 1) confirm the conclusions of the first survey concerning the prevalence and relative importance of fatigue as a side effect of cancer treatment; 2) clarify the experience of fatigue in patients; 3) further explore the impact of fatigue on the daily lives of both patients and caregivers, and 4) develop insights into how physicians can better communicate with their cancer patients. Unlike our first survey, the present survey evaluated the duration of fatigue and the economic/occupational impact of fatigue on both patients and caregivers.

Wirthlin Worldwide Research (New York, NY) was commissioned by the Fatigue Coalition to conduct a quantitative survey to further assess the effects of cancer-related fatigue during and after chemotherapy. The survey was conducted from July to August 1998. Patients were recruited from a nationally representative panel of 575,000 households in the United States (US). Households identified as having a member diagnosed with cancer were contacted by telephone; only households with a member who had undergone treatment with chemotherapy alone or with radiotherapy were eligible to participate in a 25-minute interview, which included approximately 50 questions.

Initially, patients were asked background questions about their current condition and medical history (e.g. type of cancer, side effects experienced during and after chemotherapy) and how often they had experienced fatigue (defined as a general feeling of debilitating tiredness or loss of energy). Patients who reported they "hardly ever" experienced fatigue were asked only a few additional demographic questions for statistical purposes. Those who experienced

Table 1. Patient profile (n = 379)

Demographic	Percent
Gender	
Male	21
Female	79
Age (years)	
≤ 44	8
45-54	19
55-64	26
65-74	29
≥ 75	17
Type of cancer[*]	
Breast	62
Genitourinary	12
Leukemia/lymphoma	11
Gastrointestinal	7
Gynecologic	7
Other	13
Don't know/refused	1
Type of treatment	
Chemotherapy	53%
Chemotherapy and radiotherapy	47%
Education	
Less than high school	6
High school graduate	32
Some college	30
College graduate	18
Postgraduate	13
Household income	
Less than $15,000	13
$15,000-$24,999	17
$25,000-$49,999	28
≥$50,000	24
Don't know/refused	18

[*]More than one type of cancer was an acceptable answer

fatigue at least a few days each month were asked a series of questions aimed at describing fatigue, its impact compared to the other common chemotherapy-induced side effects of nausea, pain, and depression, and the level of communication with health care professionals. Additional questions examined the impact of fatigue on daily functioning, including physical, mental/emotional, behavioral/social, and occupational/economic effects. Patients also were asked questions that examined the occupational/economic effects of their fatigue and chemotherapy regimen on primary caregivers. Types of questions addressing the impact of fatigue consisted primarily of open-ended questions and lists of statements, which were read to patients and answered with "yes" or "no" responses.

Patient population

Of the 575,000 households from the nationally representative panel, 6,125 included a patient with cancer; 406 of these households had individuals who received chemotherapy alone or with radiotherapy. Overall, 379 (93% response rate) patients were interviewed, and the sampling error was ± 6%.

Patient demographics for the 379 patients are shown in Table 1. The median patient age was 62 years. Fifty-three percent of the interviewed patients received chemotherapy only, whereas the remainder (47%) had a history of chemotherapy and radiotherapy. Forty percent of patients had their last chemotherapy treatment within the past two years, whereas 60% had been treated with chemotherapy more than two years previously.

Prevalence and duration of fatigue

When patients were asked what side effect affected them most *during* chemotherapy, nausea was most commonly identified (34%), followed by fatigue (18%) and hair loss (11%). The side effect with the greatest impact *after* completion of chemotherapy was fatigue (reported by 25% of patients; Table 2). Of the interviewed patients, 301 (76%) reported experiencing fatigue at least a few days each month during their most recent chemotherapy (Fig. 1), compared with 54% reporting nausea, 23% reporting depression, and 20% reporting pain. Thirty percent of patients reported experiencing fatigue on a daily basis; women were more likely than men to report experiencing daily fatigue (33% vs 22%, respectively).

Table 2. Side effects affecting ≥2% of patients the most after completing chemotherapy (n = 379)

Side effect	% of patients
Fatigue	25
Nausea	13
Hair loss	6
Diarrhea and/or constipation	2
Weight loss and/or gain	2
Hot flashes/menopause	2

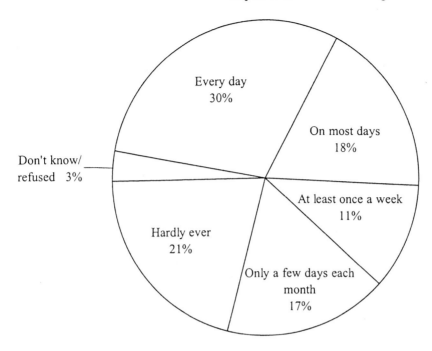

Fig. 1. Prevalence of fatigue in cancer patients (n = 379). [While undergoing your most recent treatment, how often did you feel fatigue, that is, a general feeling of debilitating tiredness or loss of energy? Would you say you felt this way every day, on most days, at least once a week, only a few days each month, or hardly ever?]

Of those who experienced fatigue during and after their most recent chemotherapy regimen, 62% and 33% said it lasted for longer than four days and two weeks, respectively. Patients over 55 years of age were more likely than younger patients (50% vs 36%, respectively) to experience fatigue that lasted longer than one week during and after their most recent chemotherapy. When patients who experienced fatigue *and* pain, nausea, or depression (n = 198) were asked which of their symptoms lasted the longest, 54% identified fatigue (Table 3).

Impact of fatigue

Physical

The majority (90%) of respondents who reported fatigue considered themselves very or somewhat active prior to being diagnosed with cancer. Physical manifestations of fatigue were most commonly described as a significantly diminished energy level (81%), need to slow down from a normal pace (81%), general

Table 3. Duration of fatigue relative to other side effects/symptoms[*]

	Symptom rank	% Rank 1st[†]	Mean score[‡]
Fatigue	1st	54	1.6
Nausea	2nd	27	2.1
Depression	3rd	12	2.5
Pain	4th	6	3.1

[*]Question: Which of these side effects or symptoms lasted the longest: pain, nausea, fatigue, or depression?

[†]Patients who experience(d) fatigue *and* pain, nausea, or depression (n = 198).

[‡]Rank based on a scale from 1 (longest) to 4 (shortest).

sense of sluggishness or tiredness (79%), and an increased need for sleep or rest (78%). When experiencing fatigue, an average of 2.8 additional hours of sleep/ rest were required per day.

Of the 301 patients who reported fatigue, 275 (91%) said it prevented them from leading a "normal" life, and 266 (88%) indicated an alteration of their daily routine due to fatigue. Sixty percent of patients who experienced fatigue and pain, nausea, or depression (n = 198) reported that fatigue affected their daily lives the most (Table 4). Specific daily activities identified as being more difficult when experiencing fatigue included walking distances, general household chores, cleaning/straightening up the house, social activities, and food preparation (Fig. 2). On average, when feeling fatigued, patients reported an ability to accomplish only 55% of activities normally performed. Subsets of patients more likely to have their daily routine substantially affected by fatigue included those who were middle-aged (aged 55-64; 60% vs 44% of younger and older patients) or active prior to diagnosis (58% vs 39% of those less active).

Table 4. Impact of fatigue on daily living relative to other side effects/symptoms[*]

	Symptom rank	% Rank 1st[†]	Mean score[‡]
Fatigue	1st	60	1.5
Nausea	2nd	22	2.1
Depression	3rd	10	2.6
Pain	4th	6	3.1

[*]Question: Which of these side effects or symptoms do you think affects/affected your everyday life more: pain, nausea, fatigue, or depression?

[†]Patients who experience(d) fatigue *and* pain, nausea, or depression (n = 198).

[‡]Rank based on a scale from 1 (greatest) to 4 (least).

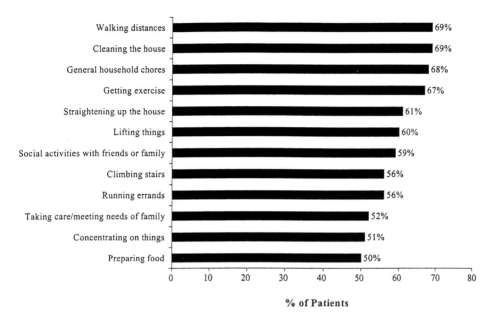

Fig. 2. Daily activities that were "a lot" or "somewhat" more difficult in ≥50% of cancer patients (n = 301) when experiencing fatigue.

Psychosocial

The mental/emotional effects of fatigue reported in ≥30% of patients are summarized in Figure 3. Most patients reported a need to push themselves to do things (77%), decreased motivation or interest (62%), and feelings of sadness, frustration, or irritability (53%) during their experiences with fatigue. In addition, fatigue affected typical cognitive tasks, such as concentrating (38%), remembering things (35%), and keeping dates straight (34%). Patients younger than 54 years were almost twice as likely as older patients to feel misunderstood (60% vs 33% of those older), depressed and hopeless (51% vs 29% of those older), and like they wanted to die (28% vs 16% of those older).

The social/behavioral activities that were more difficult in ≥30% of patients when experiencing fatigue are summarized in Figure 4. Exercise and shopping were more difficult during episodes of fatigue in 64% and 57% of patients, respectively. Fatigue also made it more difficult to participate in social activities such as going to a restaurant (35%), keeping up with interpersonal relationships (37%), and spending time with friends (35%).

Economic/occupational

Most (59%) of the 301 patients who experienced fatigue were actively working at the time of cancer diagnosis. The occupational impact of fatigue on patients

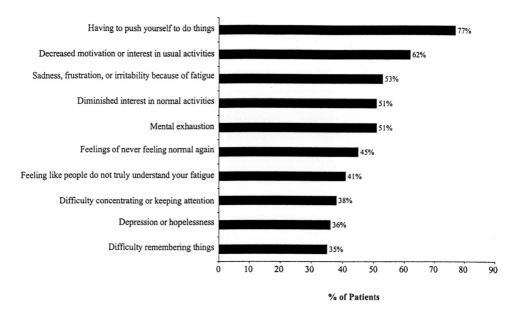

Fig. 3. Mental and emotional effects reported in ≥30% of cancer patients (n = 301) when experiencing fatigue.

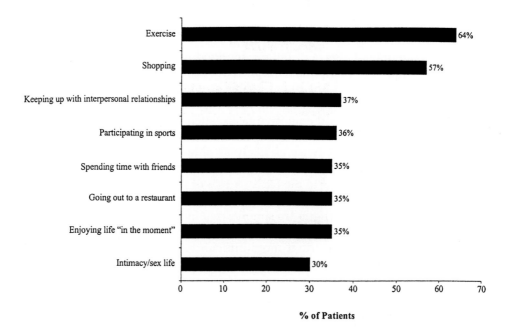

Fig. 4. Social and behavioral activities that were "a lot" or "somewhat" more difficult in ≥30% of cancer patients (n = 301) when experiencing fatigue.

and the occupational impact of the patient's cancer treatment on primary care-givers are summarized in Figure 5. Of the 177 patients who were employed, 75% changed their employment status as a result of fatigue. The mean number of sick/vacation days typically used as a result of fatigue was 4.2 per month (during and immediately after treatment). In extreme cases, patients discontinued work altogether (28%), went on disability (23%), or used unpaid family and medical leave (11%) because of fatigue (during or immediately after treatment); men were more likely than women to stop working altogether because of fatigue (43% vs 24%, respectively). Additionally, patients needed to hire help to take care of daily chores such as cleaning (22%), yard work (18%), and cooking (5%).

Patients reported that, while they were undergoing chemotherapy, their primary caregivers took more time off work (20%), accepted fewer responsibilities (18%), or reduced worked hours (11%) (Fig. 5). Twelve percent of primary caregivers had to use unpaid family leave or were forced to stop working completely. Furthermore, 65% of patients indicated that their fatigue resulted in their primary caregivers taking at least one day (mean, 4.5 days) off work in a typical month.

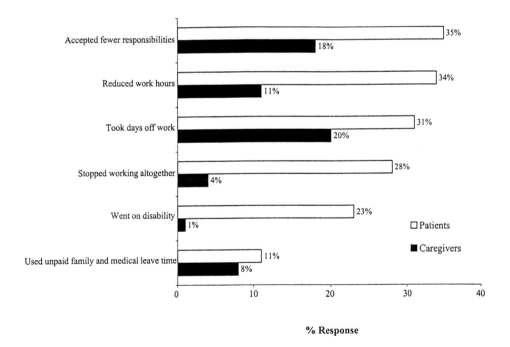

% Response

Fig. 5. Occupational effects of fatigue reported in ≥10% of cancer patients working at the time of diagnosis (n = 177) and the occupational impact of the patient's cancer treatment on primary caregivers (n = 301).

Patient-physician communication

Physicians were the health care professionals most commonly consulted to discuss fatigue (79%), followed by nurses (28%) and physicians' assistants (5%). Eight percent of patients indicated that they had never discussed their fatigue with a health care professional. Reasons for not discussing fatigue with a health care professional most often included assumptions that it was an expected outcome of their cancer treatment (79%), would not persist much longer (61%), or was caused by cancer (49%). Furthermore, 45% of patients believed that nothing could be done to relieve or reduce fatigue. Patients aged 65 years or older were least likely to discuss fatigue with health care professionals (3% vs 16% of those younger).

Management of fatigue

When asked what was recommended or prescribed for reducing fatigue, 40% of patients stated that nothing was offered (Fig. 6). Bed rest/relaxation (37%) was most commonly recommended for reducing fatigue, followed by diet or nutrition (11%), vitamins (7%), and prescription drugs (6%).

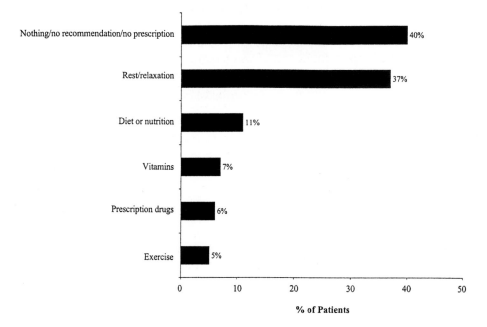

Fig. 6. Strategies for fatigue reduction that were recommended or prescribed for >1% of cancer patients (n = 301). [What, if anything, did your doctor prescribe or recommend to help reduce your fatigue?]

Discussion

This survey was designed to characterize the prevalence and duration of cancer-related fatigue and its impact from the perspective of cancer patients treated with chemotherapy alone or with radiotherapy. The fatigue prevalence rate of 76% is consistent with results of our initial survey [6] and previous studies that assessed the prevalence of fatigue in patients with cancer [1,5,12,14,15,18-21]. Fatigue was more prevalent and associated with a longer duration than other chemotherapy-induced side effects. More than 50% of patients reported that fatigue lasted longer than nausea, depression, and pain, and one third reported a duration of longer than two weeks.

The high prevalence of fatigue in cancer patients may be due in part to the evolution of more intensive treatment strategies, including combined modality approaches and high-dose chemotherapy [17]. In this survey, the chemotherapy and chemotherapy/radiotherapy groups were not evaluated separately. It is possible that inclusion of patients with a history of radiotherapy may have contributed to the long duration of fatigue, as radiotherapy-induced fatigue is often cumulative, peaking after several weeks [3,20,22-24].

Experience indicates that evaluation of fatigue in cancer patients is difficult due to the subjectivity of this measure of functional performance [25]. Therefore, explicit questions concerning common daily activities were asked in attempts to improve the objectivity of our survey. The reported effects of fatigue on daily physical and psychosocial functioning of cancer patients were substantial and consistent with results of previous studies [4,7,8,15,24,26]. Most patients who reported fatigue said it prevented them from leading a normal life and conducting their daily routine. Social activities such as going to a restaurant and spending time with friends became more difficult. Fatigue was also associated with a wide range of symptoms consistent with psychological impairment, including a lack of motivation, depression, and disturbances in mood and cognition. Although cancer-related fatigue can occur independent of physical performance level [25], the present survey suggests that patients with low physical performance levels were more depressed, anxious, and socially insecure. The correlation of fatigue with pain and depression was not investigated in the present survey; however, existing evidence suggests that these symptoms are correlated with fatigue in cancer patients [4,12,21]. The cause-and-effect relationship between psychological distress and the physical manifestations of cancer-related fatigue remains unclear and requires further investigation [13,15,18,25,27].

The ability to work is considered a concrete indicator of quality of life [28]. The reported impact of fatigue on the abilities of patients to continue working normally was substantial in the present survey. More than 75% of patients admitted changing their responsibilities because of fatigue. Furthermore, more than 20% of patients stopped working completely or went on disability. An interesting finding of our survey was the high occupational impact of the patients' cancer treatment on primary caregivers. Twelve percent of cancer patients reported that their primary caregiver was forced to take unpaid leave or stop working completely.

Our initial fatigue survey showed that fatigue was undertreated and seldom discussed among patients, caregivers, and oncologists [6]. Similarly, 40% of patients with fatigue in the present survey indicated that they were not offered any recommendations for reducing possible contributing factors or achieving symptomatic relief. The rate of discussion with health-care professionals (92%) was encouraging; however, it is important to note that 45% of patients did not discuss fatigue more often because they believed nothing could be done to relieve it. As in our initial survey, bed rest/relaxation was the most common recommendation for relieving fatigue despite the potential physical and psychologic benefits of exercise in cancer patients [25,29-32 and the chapter by V. Mock in this volume]. Although patients may benefit from correction of potential etiologies and comorbidities (e.g. pain, depression, anemia, and metabolic/nutritional abnormalities), these strategies were not pursued [2,3,16]. Further education for cancer patients, caregivers, and health care professionals on the availability of effective strategies and the development of individualized treatment plans targeted at alleviating fatigue is warranted. In addition, the importance of discussing fatigue with health care professionals should be emphasized to patients [2].

Cancer-related fatigue is common among cancer patients receiving chemotherapy with or without radiotherapy. A high percentage of these patients suffer debilitating fatigue that affects their physical and psychosocial wellbeing and ability to work. Given the substantial effect of cancer-related fatigue on quality of life, evaluation and treatment options for this symptom should routinely be considered to alleviate this condition [3].

References

1   Portenoy RK, Thaler HT, Kornblith AB, et al. Symptom prevalence, characteristics, and distress in a cancer population. Qual Life Res 1994; 3: 183-9
2   Cella D, Peterman A, Passik S, et al. Progress toward guidelines for the management of fatigue. Oncology 1998; 12: 369-77
3   Portenoy RK, Itri LM. Cancer-related fatigue: Guidelines for evaluation and management. The Oncologist 1999; 4: 1-10
4   Irvine D, Vincent L, Graydon JE, et al. The prevalence and correlates of fatigue in patients receiving treatment with chemotherapy and radiotherapy: A comparison with the fatigue experienced by healthy individuals. Cancer Nurs 1994; 17: 367-78
5   Macquart-Moulin G, Veins P, Genre D, et al. Concomitant chemoradiotherapy for patients with nonmetastatic breast carcinoma: Side effects, quality of life, and daily organization. Cancer 1999; 85: 2190-9
6   Vogelzang NJ, Breitbart W, Cella D, et al. Patient, caregiver, and oncologist perceptions of cancer-related fatigue: Results of a tripart assessment survey. Semin Hematol 1997; 34 (suppl 2): 4-12
7   Yellen SB, Cella DF, Webster K, et al. Measuring fatigue and other anemia-related symptoms with the Functional Assessment of Cancer Therapy (FACT) measurement system. J Pain Symptom Manage 1997; 13: 63-74
8   Rhodes VA, Watson PM, Hanson BM. Patients' descriptions of the influence of tiredness and weakness on self-care abilities. Cancer Nurs 1988; 11: 186-94

9   Winningham ML, Nail LM, Burke MB, et al. Fatigue and the cancer experience: The state of the knowledge. Oncol Nurs Forum 1994; 21: 23-36

10 Portenoy RK, Miaskowski C. Assessment and management of cancer-related fatigue. In: Berger A, Portenoy RK, Weissman DE, eds. Principles and practice of supportive oncology. Philadelphia: Lippincott-Raven Publishers, 1998; 109-18

11 Aistars J. Fatigue in the cancer patient: A conceptual approach to a clinical problem. Oncol Nurs Forum 1987; 14: 25-30

12 Blesch KS, Paice JA, Wickham R, et al. Correlates of fatigue in people with breast or lung cancer. Oncol Nurs Forum 1991; 18: 81-7

13 Stone P, Richards M, Hardy J. Fatigue in patients with cancer. Eur J Cancer 1998; 34: 1670-6

14 Irvine DM, Vincent L, Bubela N, et al. A critical appraisal of the research literature investigating fatigue in the individual with cancer. Cancer Nurs 1991; 14: 188-99

15 Meyerowitz BE, Sparks FC, Spears IK. Adjuvant chemotherapy for breast carcinoma: Psychosocial implications. Cancer 1979; 43: 1613-8

16 Bruera E, MacDonald RN. Asthenia in patients with advanced cancer. J Pain Symptom Manage 1988; 3: 9-14

17 Glaus A. Fatigue – an orphan topic in patients with cancer? (editorial) Eur J Cancer 1998; 34: 1649-51

18 Bruera E, Brenneis C, Michaud M, et al. Asthenia in breast cancer. Am J Nurs 1989; 89: 737, 738, 741

19 Cassileth BR, Lusk EJ, Bodenheimer BJ, et al. Chemotherapeutic toxicity – the relationship between patients' pretreatment expectations and post-treatment results. Am J Clin Oncol 1985; 8: 419-25

20 King KB, Nail LM, Kreamer K, et al. Patients' descriptions of the experience of receiving radiation therapy. Oncol Nurs Forum 1985; 12: 55-61

21 Stone P, Hardy J, Broadley K, et al. Fatigue in advanced cancer: A prospective controlled cross-sectional study. Br J Cancer 1999; 79: 1479-86

22 Greenberg DB, Sawicka J, Eisenthal S, et al. Fatigue syndrome due to localized radiation. J Pain Symptom Manage 1992; 7: 38-45

23 Haylock PJ, Hart LK. Fatigue in patients receiving localized radiation. Cancer Nurs 1979; 2: 461-7

24 Kobashi-Schoot JAM, Hanewald GJFP, Van Dam FSAM, et al. Assessment of malaise in cancer patients treated with radiotherapy. Cancer Nurs 1985; 8: 306-13

25 Dimeo FC, Tilmann MHM, Bertz H, et al. Aerobic exercise in the rehabilitation of cancer patients after high dose chemotherapy and autologous peripheral stem cell transplantation. Cancer 1997; 79: 1717-22

26 Nerenz DR, Leventhal H, Love RR. Factors contributing to emotional distress during cancer chemotherapy. Cancer 1982; 50: 1020-7

27 Visser MRM, Smets EMA. Fatigue, depression and quality of life in cancer patients: How are they related? Support Care Cancer 1998; 6: 101-8

28 Cella D. Factors influencing quality of life in cancer patients: Anemia and fatigue. Semin Oncol 1998; 25 (suppl 7): 43-6

29 Dimeo FC, Stieglitz R-D, Novelli-Fischer U, et al. Effects of physical activity on the fatigue and psychologic status of cancer patients during chemotherapy. Cancer 1999; 85: 2273-7

30 MacVicar MG, Winningham ML, Nickel JL. Effects of aerobic interval training on cancer patients' functional capacity. Nurs Res 1989; 38: 348-51

31 Mock V, Dow KH, Meares CJ, et al. Effects of exercise on fatigue, physical functioning, and emotional distress during radiation therapy for breast cancer. Oncol Nurs Forum 1997; 6: 991-1000

32 Winningham ML. Walking program for people with cancer: Getting started. Cancer Nurs 1991; 14: 270-6

APPENDIX

The Fatigue Coalition is a multidisciplinary group of medical practitioners, researchers, and patient advocates formed to develop educational and research initiatives designed to help patients, physicians, and other practitioners better understand the onset, duration, and progression of fatigue in patients with cancer or AIDS and provide successful interventions. The Fatigue Coalition is underwritten by Ortho Biotech Inc., a biotechnology subsidiary of Johnson & Johnson.

The Fatigue Coalition:

William Breitbart, Memorial Sloan-Kettering Cancer Center, New York, NY
David Cella, Evanston Northwestern Healthcare, Evanston, IL
Gregory A. Curt, National Cancer Institute, Bethesda, MD
Jerome E. Groopman, Harvard Medical School, Beth Israel Deaconess Medical Center, Boston, MA
Sandra J. Horning, Stanford University Medical Center, Stanford, CA
David H. Johnson, Vanderbilt University, Nashville, TN
Loretta M. Itri, Ortho Biotech Inc., Raritan, NJ
Christine Miaskowski, University of California San Francisco, San Francisco, CA
Russell K. Portenoy, Beth Israel Medical Center, New York, NY
Susan L. Scherr, National Coalition for Cancer Survivorship, Silver Spring, MD
Nicholas J. Vogelzang, University of Chicago, Chicago, IL

ESO Scientific Updates, Vol. 5
Fatigue and Cancer
M. Marty and S. Pecorelli, editors

Cancer-Related Fatigue: Guidelines for Evaluation and Management

Russell K. Portenoy[1] and Loretta M. Itri[2]

1   Department of Pain Medicine and Palliative Care, Beth Israel Medical Center, New York, NY, USA
2   Clinical Affairs, Ortho Biotech Products, L.P., Raritan, NJ, USA

Introduction

Fatigue has been identified by patients with cancer as a major obstacle to normal functioning and a good quality of life [1]. It is a nearly universal symptom in patients undergoing primary antineoplastic therapy or treatment with biologic response modifiers and is extremely common in populations with persistent or advanced disease [1-12].

Given the prevalence and impact of cancer-related fatigue, there have been remarkably few studies of the phenomenon. Its epidemiology has been poorly defined, and the variety of clinical presentations remains anecdotal. The existence of discrete fatigue syndromes linked with predisposing factors or potential etiologies has not been confirmed, and clinical trials to evaluate putative therapies for specific types of cancer-related fatigue are almost entirely lacking.

It is important to begin to characterize the phenomenon of cancer-related fatigue and offer guidelines for management. Increased awareness will encourage better assessment and consideration of available therapeutic options. Management will improve as new research clarifies the prevalence and nature of the problem, yields validated assessment tools, and evaluates specific treatment strategies. This review discusses the clinical aspects of cancer-related fatigue and offers strategies to assist in the management of this undertreated condition.

Adapted with permission from Portenoy RK, Itri LM. Cancer-Related Fatigue: Guidelines for Evaluation and Management. The Oncologist 1999; 4: 1-10, ©AlphaMed Press 1083-7159

Address for correspondence: R.K. Portenoy, MD, Department of Pain Medicine and Palliative Care, Beth Israel Medical Center, First Avenue at 16th Street, New York, NY 10003, USA. Tel.: +1-212-844-1505, fax: +1-212-844-1503, e-mail: RPortenoy@BethIsraelNY.org

Definition, prevalence and causes of fatigue

Patients and practitioners can generally differentiate "normal" fatigue experienced by the general population from clinical fatigue associated with cancer or its treatment. The term "asthenia" has been used to describe fatigue in oncology patients but has no specific meaning apart from the more common term. Fatigue is an inherently subjective and multidimensional condition. It may be described in terms of a variety of characteristics (e.g. severity, distress, temporal features) and specific impairments (e.g. lack of energy, weakness, somnolence, difficulty concentrating). Criteria have been needed to define this clinically relevant syndrome. Recently, cancer-related fatigue was accepted as a diagnosis in the International Classification of Diseases 10th Revision-Clinical Modification. Fatigue may be characterized as a multidimensional phenomenon that develops over time, diminishing energy, mental capacity, and the psychologic condition of cancer patients (Table 1) [13]. Fatigue is also linked with lethargy, malaise, and asthenia in the revised National Cancer Institute (NCI) Common Toxicity Criteria (CTC). These classifications may enhance awareness of fatigue and improve reporting of the condition.

Table 1. Proposed criteria for cancer-related fatigue [13]

The following symptoms have been present every day or nearly every day during the same two-week period in the past month:

- Significant fatigue, diminished energy, or increased need to rest, disproportionate to any recent change in activity level

Plus five (or more) of the following:

- Complaints of generalized weakness or limb heaviness
- Diminished concentration or attention
- Decreased motivation or interest in engaging in usual activities
- Insomnia or hypersomnia
- Experience of sleep as unrefreshing or nonrestorative
- Perceived need to struggle to overcome inactivity
- Marked emotional reactivity (e.g. sadness, frustration, or irritability) to feeling fatigued
- Difficulty completing daily tasks attributed to feeling fatigued
- Perceived problems with short-term memory
- Post-exertional malaise lasting several hours

The symptoms cause clinically significant distress or impairment in social, occupational, or other important areas of functioning.

There is evidence from the history, physical examination, or laboratory findings that the symptoms are a consequence of cancer or cancer-related therapy.

The symptoms are not primarily a consequence of comorbid psychiatric disorders such as major depression, somatization disorder, somatoform disorder, or delirium.

Cancer-related fatigue is extremely prevalent. A recent population-based survey of 419 randomly selected patients observed that 78% experienced fatigue, which was defined as debilitating tiredness or loss of energy at least once each week; the majority of these patients reported that fatigue had either significantly (31%) or somewhat (39%) affected their daily routine [1]. In a cross-sectional survey of 151 ovarian cancer patients, the prevalence of fatigue was 69%, and approximately half of affected patients described the condition as highly distressing [11]. Other surveys of patients with metastatic disease suggest that the prevalence in this setting exceeds 75% [11,14-18].

Numerous surveys have associated the occurrence of fatigue with specific treatments [3-6,19-23]. These surveys suggest that fatigue commonly occurs after surgery, chemotherapy, radiotherapy, or immunotherapy. Prevalence rates of fatigue as high as 96% have been reported in conjunction with chemotherapy and radiotherapy [5], and severe fatigue is almost universal with the use of biologic response modifiers, including alpha-interferon and the interleukins [19,23, 24].

When fatigue is primarily related to a treatment, there is generally a clear temporal relationship between the condition and the intervention [21,25-27]. In patients receiving cyclic chemotherapy, for example, fatigue often peaks within a few days and declines until the next treatment cycle. During a course of fractionated radiotherapy, fatigue is often cumulative and may peak after a period of weeks. Occasionally, fatigue persists for a prolonged period beyond the end of chemotherapy or radiotherapy.

The relationships between fatigue and demographic characteristics, physiologic factors, and psychosocial factors are not well defined. The specific mechanisms that precipitate or sustain the syndrome are unknown. Fatigue may represent a final common pathway to which many predisposing or etiologic factors contribute (Table 2) [29-35]. The pathophysiology in any individual may be multifactorial. Proposed mechanisms include abnormalities in energy metabolism related to increased requirements (e.g. due to tumor growth, infection, fever, or surgery); decreased availability of metabolic substrate (e.g. due to anemia, hypoxemia, or poor nutrition); or the abnormal production of substances that impair metabolism or normal functioning of muscles (e.g. cytokines or antibodies). Other proposed mechanisms link fatigue to the pathophysiology of sleep disorders and major depression. There is no clear evidence in support of any of these mechanisms, and further research is needed.

Evaluation of fatigue

Assessment of fatigue characteristics

A detailed characterization of fatigue, coupled with an understanding of the most likely etiologic factors, is necessary to develop a therapeutic strategy (Table 3). A comprehensive assessment includes a description of fatigue-related

Table 2. Potential predisposing factors or etiologies of cancer-related fatigue [28]

Physiologic	Psychosocial
Underlying disease	*Anxiety disorders*
Treatment for the disease	*Depressive disorders*
Chemotherapy	
Radiotherapy	*Stress*
Surgery	
Biologic response modifiers	*Environmental reinforcers*
Intercurrent systemic disorders	
Anemia	
Infection	
Pulmonary disorders	
Hepatic failure	
Heart failure	
Renal insufficiency	
Malnutrition	
Neuromuscular disorders	
Dehydration or electrolyte disturbances	
Sleep disorders	
Immobility and lack of exercise	
Chronic pain	
Use of centrally acting drugs (e.g. opioids)	

Table 3. Evaluation of cancer-related fatigue

Assessment of fatigue characteristics and manifestations

Severity, temporal features (onset, course, duration, daily pattern), exacerbating and palliative factors, associated distress, impact

Lack of energy, muscle weakness, somnolence, dysphoric mood, or impaired cognitive function

Evaluation of potential etiologies and comorbid conditions

Evaluation of broader constructs

Quality of life, symptom distress, goals of care

phenomena, a physical examination, and a review of laboratory and imaging studies. These data may allow plausible hypotheses concerning pathogenesis, which in turn may suggest appropriate treatment strategies.

Patients may describe fatigue in terms of decreased vitality or lack of energy, muscular weakness, dysphoric mood, somnolence, impaired cognitive functioning, or some combination of these disturbances. Although this variability suggests the existence of fatigue subtypes, this has not yet been empirically confirmed. Regardless, the patient's history should clarify the spectrum of complaints and attempt to characterize features associated with each component. This information may suggest specific etiologies (e.g. depression) and influence the choice of therapy. Neurologic and psychologic evaluations also may help further clarify potential etiologies of fatigue in some patients.

Other characteristics are similarly important. Onset and duration, for example, distinguish acute and chronic fatigue. Acute fatigue has a recent onset and is anticipated to end in the near future. Chronic fatigue has persisted for a prolonged period (weeks to months, or longer) and is not expected to remit soon. Patients perceived to have chronic fatigue typically require a more intensive evaluation, as well as a management approach focused on both short- and long-term goals. Other important descriptors of fatigue include its severity, daily pattern, course over time, exacerbating and palliative factors, and associated distress.

To measure fatigue severity, consistent use of a simple unidimensional scale, such as a verbal rating scale (none, mild, moderate, severe) or a numeric scale (for example, a 0-10 scale, where "0" equals no fatigue and "10" equals the worst fatigue imaginable, or a 0-4 scale, as applied in the NCI CTC) are useful for monitoring changes over time [36]. Other unidimensional scales include the fatigue subscale of the Profile of Mood States [37], linear analog scales (linear analog scale assessment [LASA]) [38], and single items incorporated into symptom checklists [39-41].

Multidimensional fatigue assessment, which captures multiple characteristics and manifestations of fatigue and its impact on function, is more informative than the measurement of severity alone. In the practice setting, when time for evaluation is limited, the routine use of three simple questions may help assess fatigue severity and impact over time [36]:
- Are you experiencing any fatigue?
- If yes, how severe has it been, on average, during the past week, using a 0-10 scale?
- How is the fatigue interfering with your ability to function?

Validated multidimensional questionnaires provide a more sophisticated alternative for practice, or, more commonly, for use in research settings [12,22,36, 42-47].

Multidimensional assessment tools

The first validated multidimensional instrument was the Piper Fatigue Self-Report Scale. This scale addresses the severity, distress, and impact of fatigue using a 41-item questionnaire administered as either a series of LASA or numeric scales [36]. It was developed to assess fatigue in patients receiving radiotherapy. It is both reliable and valid in this population and may also be used to assess cancer patients who are not receiving radiotherapy. Efforts continue to further refine it [48].

A 20-item scale that evaluates well-being associated with fatigue and anemia has been developed as a module of a general quality of life instrument known as the Functional Assessment of Cancer Therapy (FACT) [12,42,43]. The fatigue, or fatigue and anemia, subscales of this module can be used alone as brief, reliable, and valid assessments. Using this questionnaire, an association between fatigue and anemia was demonstrated in a large survey of cancer patients in community settings. Patients with hemoglobin values >12 g/dl reported significantly less fatigue, fewer nonfatigue anemia symptoms, better physical and functional well-being, and a higher overall quality of life than those with hemoglobin values ≤12 g/dl [49].

Other validated multidimensional instruments are available [9,44-47]. The Fatigue Symptom Inventory, for example, has been used in a series of studies that evaluated the severity and impact of treatment-related fatigue [44]. Investigators or clinicians who seek a detailed assessment of fatigue should review the items in these questionnaires and select the instrument that captures the fatigue-related phenomena of greatest interest.

Assessment of related constructs

An assessment of cancer-related fatigue also should include consideration of broader concerns, including global quality of life, symptom distress, and the goals of care. Fatigue may be only one of numerous factors that influence quality of life. Among these factors are progressive physical decline, psychological disorders, social isolation, financial concerns, and spiritual distress. Optimal care of the cancer patient includes a broad assessment of these factors and should be directed toward maintaining or enhancing quality of life.

The concept of global symptom distress is useful in characterizing patients who often have multiple symptoms concurrently [39-41]. Fatigue, pain, and psychological distress are the most prevalent symptoms across varied cancer populations [41]. Patients who report fatigue should be queried about the presence of other symptoms and the degree to which fatigue predominates as a cause of distress.

The goals of care guide all therapeutic decision making. Specific treatments may or may not be appropriate depending on the degree to which the preeminent goals relate to prolonging life, improving function, or providing comfort alone.

Management strategies

A successful strategy should ameliorate fatigue within a broader approach to patient care. Education of the patient regarding the nature of fatigue, options for therapy, and anticipated outcomes is an essential aspect of the therapy. Unfortunately, results of a recent survey indicate that fatigue is seldom discussed by patients and their oncologists [1].

Treatment of underlying causes

As an initial approach to cancer-related fatigue, efforts should be made to correct potential etiologies, if possible and appropriate (Fig. 1). This may include elimination of nonessential centrally-acting drugs, treatment of a sleep disorder, reversal of anemia or metabolic abnormalities, or management of major depression. Many of these initial interventions are relatively simple and pose minimal burdens to the patient, healthcare provider, and caregiver.

In patients with fatigue associated with major depression, treatment with an antidepressant is strongly indicated. As many as 25% of cancer patients develop major depression at some point during the illness; patients at greatest risk are those with advanced disease, uncontrolled physical symptoms (e.g. pain), or previous history of psychiatric disorder [50]. Although the relationship between depression and fatigue is not understood, they often occur together, and both adversely affect quality of life [51,52]. Despite the high prevalence in the cancer population, depression is often underdiagnosed, and, consequently, undertreated [53,54]. A trial with an antidepressant usually is warranted in a patient with fatigue associated with any significant degree of depressed mood, particularly if concurrent anxiety or pain exists.

Anemia may be a major factor in the development of cancer-related fatigue. Anecdotally, transfusion therapy for severe anemia often has been associated with substantial improvement in fatigue. Until the early 1980s, red blood cell transfusions were administered empirically when hemoglobin concentrations fell below 10 g/dl [55,56] and were the primary treatment for cancer-related and chemotherapy-induced anemia. At that time, concern about the safety of the blood supply related to potential transmission of the human immunodeficiency virus prompted clinicians to alter their treatment approach [56,57]. Without an alternative to transfusion, treatment of mild or moderate anemia was generally avoided until hemoglobin concentrations declined to more severe levels (7-8 g/dl) or the patient experienced signs and symptoms of severe anemia [55,58]. As reticence to treat anemia increased, it was less often reported as an adverse sequela in published chemotherapy trials and received less attention in the medical literature overall.

New data demonstrate an association between chemotherapy-induced mild-to-moderate anemia and both fatigue and quality-of-life impairment. For example, combined data from 413 patients in three randomized, placebo-controlled trials of epoetin alfa, the recombinant form of human erythropoietin,

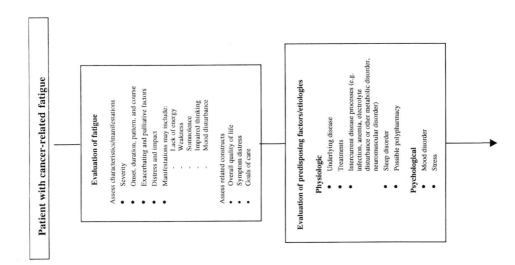

Fig. 1. Algorithm for the evaluation of cancer-related fatigue.

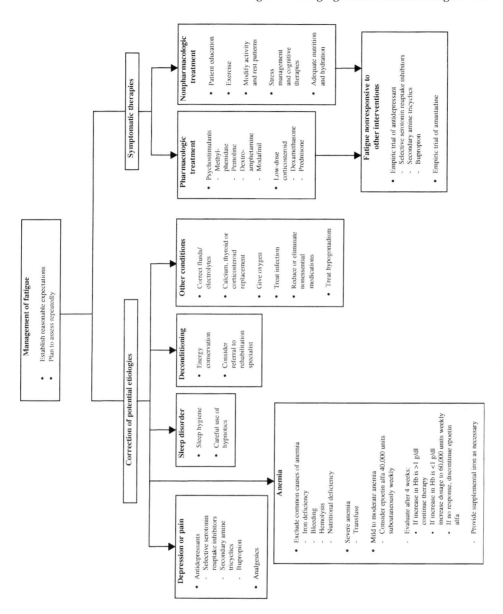

reveal that treated patients experienced a significant increase in hematocrit, a reduced need for transfusion, and a significant improvement in overall quality of life. Those patients with an increase in hematocrit of >6% also demonstrated significant improvement in energy level and daily activities [59]. Additional studies in patients treated with chemotherapy and radiation therapy for a variety of hematologic and solid tumors confirm that epoetin alfa has positive effects on hemoglobin levels [60,63].

Two large, prospective, nonrandomized, multicenter community trials evaluated the effectiveness of epoetin alfa in anemia associated with cancer chemotherapy [64,65]. In the more recent trial, Demetri et al. assessed the effectiveness of epoetin alfa as an adjunct to chemotherapy in more than 2,000 cancer patients undergoing cytotoxic chemotherapy [64]. Patients received epoetin alfa 10,000 units three times weekly for a maximum of 16 weeks. If the increase in hemoglobin level was <1.0 g/dl at four weeks, the dose was increased to 20,000 units three times weekly. Quality-of-life parameters were assessed with LASA and the FACT-Anemia instruments. Over time, patients experienced significant improvements in energy level, activity level, functional status, and overall quality of life; these improvements were independent of antitumor response and were significantly correlated with hemoglobin levels. These results were similar to the findings in the previous large, community-based study by Glaspy et al. [65].

Symptomatic approaches

Pharmacologic treatments

The pharmacologic therapies for fatigue associated with medical illness have not been rigorously evaluated in controlled trials. Nonetheless, there is evidence to support the use of several drug classes. Psychostimulants, such as methylphenidate, pemoline, and dextroamphetamine, have been well studied for the treatment of opioid-related somnolence and cognitive impairment [66], and depression in the elderly and medically ill [67-69]. There are no controlled studies of these drugs for cancer-related fatigue, but empiric administration may yield favorable results in some patients. A newer psychostimulant, modafinil, is also being used empirically.

Clinical response to one drug does not necessarily predict response to the others, and sequential trials may be needed to identify the most beneficial therapy. Methylphenidate has been more extensively evaluated in the cancer population than other stimulant drugs and often is the first drug administered. Pemoline has less sympathomimetic activity than other psychostimulants but has a low risk of severe hepatotoxicity compared with similar agents [70]. It is available in a chewable formulation that can be absorbed through the buccal mucosa for patients who are unable to swallow or take oral medications.

Adverse effects associated with the psychostimulants include anorexia, insomnia, tremulousness, anxiety, delirium, and tachycardia. To ensure safety, slow and careful dose escalation should be undertaken to minimize potential adverse effects. A regimen of methylphenidate, for example, usually begins with a dose of 5-10 mg once or twice daily (morning and, if needed, midday). If tolerated, the dose is increased. Most patients appear to require less than 60 mg per day, but some require much higher doses.

Extensive anecdotal observations and very limited data from controlled trials [71,72] support the use of low-dose corticosteroids in fatigued patients with advanced disease and multiple symptoms. Dexamethasone and prednisone are most commonly used. There have been no comparative trials.

The selective serotonin-reuptake inhibitors, secondary amine tricyclics (e.g. nortriptyline and desipramine), or bupropion are sometimes associated with the experience of increased energy that appears disproportionate to any change in mood. For this reason, these agents also have been tried empirically in non-depressed patients with fatigue. Given the limited experience in the use of these drugs for this indication, an empiric trial should be considered only in severe and refractory cases.

Amantadine has been used to treat fatigue in patients with multiple sclerosis, but it has not been studied in other patient populations. This drug is usually well tolerated, and an empiric trial may be warranted in selected patients with severe refractory cancer-related fatigue.

Nonpharmacologic interventions

Nonpharmacologic approaches for the management of cancer-related fatigue are largely supported by favorable anecdotal experience (Table 4). Patient preferences should be considered in the selection of one or more of these approaches.

Education about fatigue greatly benefits some patients [73-77]. There are large individual differences in patients' preferences for information, however, and efforts to educate should be directed at the patients' educational level and readiness to learn. The use of a patient diary may help the clinician and patient discern a pattern to the fatigue or identify specific activities that are associated with increased levels. This information may be useful in developing a management plan that modifies specific activities and incorporates appropriate periods of rest [27]. For example, some patients identify a pattern that suggests the utility of scheduled brief rest periods during the day.

Some patients benefit from education about sleep hygiene. Sleep hygiene principles should be tailored to the individual patient and might include the establishment of a specific bedtime and wake time, and routine procedures prior to sleep [78]. Patients also should be instructed to avoid stimulants and central nervous system depressants prior to sleep [78]. Regular exercise performed at least six hours before bedtime may improve sleep, whereas napping in the late afternoon or evening may worsen it.

Table 4. Nonpharmacologic interventions for the management of cancer-related fatigue

---

Patient education
  Consider the patients's preferences, education level, and readiness to learn
  Use of a patient diary

Exercise
  Individualize exercise program
  Use of rhythmic and repetitive types of exercise
  Initiate gradually

Modification of activity and rest patterns
  Assess sleep hygiene
  Establish routine sleep patterns
  Avoid use of stimulants prior to sleep
  Regular exercise

Stress management and cognitive therapies
  Use of stress reduction techniques or cognitive therapies
  Use of relaxation therapy, hypnosis, or distraction

Adequate nutrition and hydration
  Proper diet
  Monitor weight and hydration status regularly
  Referral to a dietician

Exercise may be beneficial in relieving fatigue [25,77,79-81]. This may be counterintuitive to patients, and considerable education may be needed to foster cooperation with an exercise program. There are no data that clarify the most appropriate exercise program for cancer patients with fatigue. In general, exercise should be individualized, considering such factors as the patient's age and medical condition. Anecdotally, the type of exercise that appears to be most beneficial involves rhythmic and repetitive movement of large muscle groups such as walking, cycling, or swimming. The exercise program should be initiated gradually and should include a light-to-moderate workout several days a week.

Anxiety, difficulties in coping with cancer or its treatment, or sleep disturbances may contribute to fatigue and may be ameliorated using stress reduction techniques or cognitive therapies, such as relaxation therapy, hypnosis, guided imagery, or distraction. Some patients find distraction (e.g. listening to music) or other cognitive techniques to be particularly effective when the symptom is associated with attention deficits [82,83]. Referral to a psychologist for counseling and training in stress management techniques or cognitive therapies may be warranted in some patients.

Cancer and its treatment also can interfere with dietary intake. With aggressive approaches to management, patients' weight, hydration status, and electrolyte balance should be monitored and maintained to the extent possible

[84]. Regular exercise may improve appetite and increase nutritional intake. Referral to a dietitian for nutritional guidance and suggestions for nutritional supplements may be useful.

Summary

Despite the high prevalence and distress associated with fatigue, there have been few studies of this condition, and relatively little is known about its epidemiology, etiologies, pathogenesis, and management. With growing interest in palliative care, however, there is recognition of fatigue as an important issue for research and treatment guideline development [13]. Oncologists, as well as the entire medical team, must become more aware of this problem, its impact on patient quality of life, and the various strategies that may be helpful in its treatment. Although further research is needed, many patients could benefit from a more comprehensive evaluation and greater use of available interventions for cancer-related fatigue.

References

1 Vogelzang N, Breitbart W, Cella D, et al. Patient, caregiver, and oncologist perceptions of cancer-related fatigue: results of a tripart assessment survey. Semin Hematol 1997; 34 (suppl 2): 4-12
2 Cassileth BR, Lusk EJ, Bodenheimer BJ, et al. Chemotherapeutic toxicity – the relationship between patients' pretreatment expectations and post-treatment results. Am J Clin Oncol 1985; 8: 419-25
3 Greenberg DB, Sawicka J, Eisenthal S, et al. Fatigue syndrome due to localized radiation. J Pain Symptom Manage 1992; 7: 38-45
4 Haylock PJ, Hart LK. Fatigue in patients receiving localized radiation. Cancer Nurs 1979; 2: 461-7
5 Irvine DM, Vincent L, Bubela N, et al. A critical appraisal of the research literature investigating fatigue in the individual with cancer. Cancer Nurs 1991; 14: 188-99
6 Irvine D, Vincent L, Graydon JE, et al. The prevalence and correlates of fatigue in patients receiving treatment with chemotherapy and radiotherapy: a comparison with the fatigue experienced by healthy individuals. Cancer Nurs 1994; 17: 367-78
7 King KB, Nail LM, Kreamer K, et al. Patients' descriptions of the experience of receiving radiation therapy. Oncol Nurs Forum 1985; 12: 55-61
8 Knobf MT. Physical and psychologic distress associated with adjuvant chemotherapy in women with breast cancer. J Clin Oncol 1986; 4: 678-84
9 Kobashi-Schoot JAM, Hanewald GJFP, van Dam FSAM, et al. Assessment of malaise in cancer treated with radiotherapy. Cancer Nurs 1985; 8: 306-14
10 Meyerowitz BE, Sparks FC, Spears IK. Adjuvant chemotherapy for breast carcinoma: psychosocial implications. Cancer 1979; 43: 1613-8
11 Portenoy RK, Thaler HT, Kornblith AB, et al. Pain in ovarian cancer: prevalence, characteristics, and associated symptoms. Cancer 1994; 74: 907-15
12 Yellen SB, Cella DF, Webster MA, et al. Measuring fatigue and other anemia-related symptoms with the Functional Assessment of Cancer Therapy (FACT) measurement system. J Pain Symptom Manage 1997; 13: 63-74

13 Cella D, Peterman A, Passik S, et al. Progress toward guidelines for the management of fatigue. Oncology 1998; 12: 1-9

14 Curtis EB, Kretch R, Walsh TD. Common symptoms in patients with advanced cancer. J Palliat Care 1991; 7: 25-9

15 Dunphy KP, Amesbury BDW. A comparison of hospice and homecare patients: patterns of referral, patient characteristics and predictors of place of death. Palliat Med 1990; 4: 105-11

16 Dunlop GM. A study of the relative frequency and importance of gastrointestinal symptoms and weakness in patients with far-advanced cancer: student paper. Palliat Med 1989; 4: 37-43

17 Portenoy RK, Thaler HT, Kornblith AB, et al. Symptom prevalence, characteristics, and distress in a cancer population. Qual Life Res 1994; 3: 183-9

18 Ventafridda V, DeConno F, Ripamonti C, et al. Quality of life assessment during a palliative care program. Ann Oncol 1990; 1: 415-20

19 Dean GE, Spears L, Ferrell B, et al. Fatigue in patients with cancer receiving interferon alpha. Cancer Pract 1995; 3: 164-71

20 Fobair P, Hoppe RT, Bloom J, et al. Psychosocial problems among survivors of Hodgkin's disease. J Clin Oncol 1986; 4: 805-14

21 Pickard-Holley S. Fatigue in cancer patients: a descriptive study. Cancer Nurs 1991; 14: 13-9

22 Piper BF, Lindsey AM, Dodd MJ, et al. The development of an instrument to measure the subjective dimension of fatigue. In: Funk SG, Tornquist EM, Champange MT, et al, eds. Key aspects of comfort. Management of pain, fatigue and nausea. New York: Springer Publishing Company, 1989; 199-208

23 Skalla K, Rieger P. Fatigue. In: Rieger PT, ed. Biotherapy: Comprehensive review. Boston: Jones and Bartlett, 1995; 221-42

24 Piper BF, Rieger PT, Brophy L, et al. Recent advances in the management of biotherapy-related side effects: fatigue. Oncol Nurs Forum 1989; 16 (suppl 6): 27-34

25 Berger AM. Patterns of fatigue and activity and rest during adjuvant breast cancer chemotherapy. Oncol Nurs Forum 1998; 25: 51-62

26 Broeckel JA, Jacobsen PB, Horton J, et al. Characteristics and correlates of fatigue after adjuvant chemotherapy for breast cancer. J Clin Oncol 1998; 16: 1689-96

27 Richardson A, Ream E, Wilson-Barnett J. Fatigue in patients receiving chemotherapy: patterns of change. Cancer Nurs 1998; 21: 17-30

28 Portenoy RK, Miaskowski C. Assessment and management of cancer-related fatigue. In: Berger A, Portenoy RK, Weissman DE, eds. Principles and practice of supportive oncology. Philadelphia: Lippincott-Raven, 1998; 109-18

29 Aistars J. Fatigue in the cancer patient: a conceptual approach to a clinical problem. Oncol Nurs Forum 1987; 14: 25-30

30 Piper BF, Lindsey AM, Dodd MJ. Fatigue mechanisms in cancer patients: developing nursing theory. Oncol Nurs Forum 1987; 14: 17-23

31 Jacobs LA, Piper BF. The phenomenon of fatigue and the cancer patient. In: McCorkle R, Grant M, Frank-Stromberg M, et al., eds. Cancer nursing: A comprehensive textbook. Philadelphia: WB Saunders, 1996; 1193-210

32 Nail LM, Winningham M. Fatigue. In: Groenwald SL, Frogge MH, Goodman M, et al, eds. Cancer nursing: Principles and practice. Boston: Jones and Bartlett, 1993; 608-19

33 Piper BF. Alterations in comfort: fatigue. In: McNally JC, Somerville E, Miaskowski C, et al, eds. Guidelines for oncology nursing practice, 2nd ed. Philadelphia: WB Saunders, 1991; 155-62

34 Smets EMA, Garssen B, Schuster-Uitterhoeve ALJ, et al. Fatigue in cancer patients. Br J Cancer 1993; 68: 220-4

35 Winningham ML, Nail LM, Burke MB, et al. Fatigue and the cancer experience: the state of the knowledge. Oncol Nurs Forum 1994; 21: 23-35

36 Piper BF. The Groopman article reviewed. Oncology 1998; 12: 345-6

37 Cella DF, Jacobsen PB, Orav EJ, et al. A brief POMS measure of distress for cancer patients. J Chronic Dis 1987; 40: 939-42

38 Bruera E, Chadwick S, Brenneis C, et al. Methylphenidate associated with narcotics for the treatment of cancer pain. Cancer Treat Rep 1987; 71: 67-70

39 de Haes JCJM, van Kippenberg FCE, Neijt JP. Measuring psychological and physical distress in cancer patients: structure and application of the Rotterdam Symptom Checklist. Br J Cancer 1990; 62: 1034-8

40 McCorkle R, Young K. Development of a symptom distress scale. Cancer Nurs 1978; 1: 373-8

41 Portenoy RK, Thaler HT, Kornblith AB, et al. The Memorial Symptom Assessment Scale: an instrument for the evaluation of symptom prevalence, characteristics, and distress. Eur J Cancer 1994; 30A: 1326-36

42 Cella DF, Tulsky DS, Gray G, et al. The Functional Assessment of Cancer Therapy scale: development and validation of the general measure. J Clin Oncol 1993; 11: 570-9

43 Cella D. The Functional Assessment of Cancer Therapy-Anemia (FACT-An) scale: a new tool for the assessment of outcomes in cancer anemia and fatigue. Semin Hematol 1997; 34 (suppl 2): 13-9

44 Hann DM, Jacobsen PB, Azzarello LM, et al. Measurement of fatigue in cancer patients: development and validation of the Fatigue Symptom Inventory. Qual Life Res 1998; 7: 301-10

45 Lee KA, Hicks G, Nino-Murcia G. Validity and reliability of a scale to assess fatigue. Psychiatry Res 1991; 36: 291-8

46 Morant R, Stiefel F, Berchtold W, et al. Preliminary results of a study assessing asthenia and related psychological and biological phenomena in patients with advanced cancer. Support Care Cancer 1993; 1: 101-7

47 Cleeland CC. Brief Fatigue Inventory (BFI). URL: http://www.qlmed.org/BFI/index.html

48 Piper BF, Dibble SL, Dodd MJ, et al. The revised Piper Fatigue Scale: psychometric evaluation in women in breast cancer. Oncol Nurs Forum 1998; 25: 677-84

49 Cella D. Factors influencing quality of life in cancer patients: anemia and fatigue. Semin Oncol 1998; 25: 43-6

50 Breitbart W. Identifying patients at risk for, and treatment of major psychiatric complications of cancer. Support Care Cancer 1995; 3: 45-60

51 Visser MR, Smets EM. Fatigue, depression and quality of life in cancer patients: how are they related? Support Care Cancer 1998; 6: 101-8

52 Dimeo F, Stieglitz RD, Novelli-Fischer U, et al. Correlation between physical performance and fatigue in cancer patients. Ann Oncol 1997; 8: 1251-5

53 Hardman A, Maguire P, Crowther D, et al. The recognition of psychiatric morbidity on a medical oncology ward. J Psychosom Res 1989; 33: 235-9

54 Passik SD, Dugan W, McDonald MV, et al. Oncologists' recognition of depression in their patients with cancer. J Clin Oncol 1998; 16: 1594-600

55 Consensus conference. Perioperative red cell transfusion. JAMA 1988; 260: 2700-3

56 Welch HG, Meehan KR, Goodnough LT. Prudent strategies for elective red blood cell transfusion. Ann Intern Med 1992; 116: 393-402

57 Surgenor DM, Wallace EL, Hale SG, et al. Changing patterns of blood transfusions in four sets of United States hospitals, 1980 to 1985. Transfusion 1988; 28: 513-8

58 Silberstein LE, Kruskall MS, Stehling LC, et al. Strategies for the review of transfusion practices. JAMA 1989; 262: 1993-7

59 Abels RI, Larholt KM, Drantz KD, et al. Recombinant human erythropoietin (r-Hu-EPO) for the treatment of the anemia of cancer. In: Murphy MJ, ed. Blood cell growth factors: Their present and future use in hematology and oncology. Dayton: AlphaMed Press, 1992; 121-41

60 Cascinu S, Fedeli A, Del Ferro E, et al. Recombinant human erythropoietin treatment in cisplatin-associated anemia: a randomized, double-blind trial with placebo. J Clin

Oncol 1994; 12: 1058-62

61   Ludwig H, Fritz E, Kotzmann H, et al. Erythropoietin treatment of anemia associated with multiple myeloma. N Engl J Med 1990; 322: 1693-9

62   Oster W, Hermann F, Gamm H, et al. Erythropoietin for the treatment of anemia of malignancy associated with neoplastic bone marrow infiltration. J Clin Oncol 1990; 8: 956-62

63   Platanias LC, Miller CB, Mick R, et al. Treatment of chemotherapy-induced anemia with recombinant human erythropoietin. J Clin Oncol 1991; 9: 2021-6

64   Demetri GD, Kris M, Wade J, et al. Quality-of-life benefit in chemotherapy patients treated with epoetin alfa is independent of disease response or tumor type: results from a prospective community oncology study. J Clin Oncol 1998; 16: 3412-25

65   Glaspy J, Bukowski R, Steinberg D, et al. The impact of therapy with epoetin alfa on clinical outcomes during cancer chemotherapy in community oncology practice. J Clin Oncol 1997; 15: 1218-34

66   Bruera E, Brenneis C, Paterson A, et al. Use of methylphenidate as an adjuvant to narcotic analgesics in patients with advanced cancer. J Pain Symptom Manage 1989; 4: 3-6

67   Breitbart W, Mermelstein H. An alternative psychostimulant for the management of depressive disorders in cancer patients. Psychosomatics 1992; 33: 352-6

68   Fernandez F, Adams F, Levy JK. Cognitive impairment due to AIDS-related complex and its response to psychostimulants. Psychosomatics 1988; 29: 38-46

69   Katon W, Raskind M. Treatment of depression in the medically ill elderly with methylphenidate. Am J Psychiatry 1980; 137: 963-5

70   Berkovitch M, Pope E, Phillips J, et al. Pemoline-associated fulminant liver failure: testing the evidence for causation. Clin Pharm Ther 1995; 57: 696-8

71   Bruera E, Roca E, Cedaro L, et al. Action of oral methylprednisolone in terminal cancer patients: a prospective randomized double-blind study. Cancer Treat Rep 1985; 69: 751-4

72   Tannock I, Gospodarowicz M, Meakin W, et al. Treatment of metastatic prostatic cancer with low-dose prednisone: evaluation of pain and quality of life as pragmatic indices of response. J Clin Oncol 1989; 7: 590-7

73   Egbert LD, Battit GE, Welch CE, et al. Reduction of postoperative pain by encouragement and instruction of patients. N Engl J Med 1964; 207: 825-7

74   Fortin F, Kirouac S. A randomized controlled trial of preoperative patient education. Int J Nurs Stud 1976; 13: 11-24

75   Johnson J, Fuller S, Endress MP, et al. Altering patients' responses to surgery: an extension and replication. Res Nurs Health 1978; 1: 111-21

76   Johnson J, Rice V, Fuller S, et al. Sensory information, instruction in a coping strategy, and recovery from surgery. Res Nurs Health 1978; 1: 4-17

77   Winningham ML. Fatigue. In: Groenwald SL, Frogge MH, Goodman M, et al, eds. Cancer symptom management. Boston: Jones and Bartlett, 1996; 42-58

78   Yellen SB, Dyonzak JV. Sleep disturbances. In: Groenwald SL, Frogge MH, Goodman M, et al, eds. Cancer symptom management. Boston: Jones and Bartlett, 1996; 151-68

79   Dimeo F, Rumberger BG, Keul J. Aerobic exercise as therapy for cancer fatigue. Med Sci Sports Exercise 1998; 30: 475-8

80   MacVicar SB, Winningham ML. Promoting functional capacity of cancer patients. Cancer Bull 1986; 38: 235-9

81   Schwartz AL. Patterns of exercise and fatigue in physically active cancer survivors. Oncol Nurs Forum 1998; 25: 485-91

82   Cimprich B. Attentional fatigue following breast cancer surgery. Res Nurs Health 1992; 15: 199-207

83   Cimprich B. Developing an intervention to restore attention in cancer patients. Cancer Nurs 1993; 16: 83-92

84   Dalakas MC, Mock V, Hawkins MJ. Fatigue: definitions, mechanisms, and paradigms for study. Semin Oncol 1998; 25 (suppl 1): 48-53

ESO Scientific Updates, Vol. 5
Fatigue and Cancer
M. Marty and S. Pecorelli, editors
© 2001 Elsevier Science B.V. All rights reserved

Factors Related to Fatigue in Cancer Patients: The Key to Specific Therapeutic Approaches

Michel Marty[1], Naima Bedairia[1], Valérie Laurence[2], Marc Espie[2] and Paul-Henri Cottu[2]

1   Institut Gustave Roussy, Villejuif, France
2   Département d'Oncologie Médicale, Hôpital Saint Louis, Paris, France

Introduction

While it has been known for a long time that there is a high incidence of fatigue among cancer patients, surprisingly few specific studies have been dedicated to this subject in the past. With the increasing recognition of cancer- and/ or treatment-related symptoms and the emergence of symptomatic care as an important aspect of cancer patient support, pathophysiological, grading and therapeutic studies on fatigue are now being conducted. The incidence of fatigue has been defined with more precision: it depends on the stage of cancer, on specific site/organ involvement, but also on the therapeutic modalities used.

Fatigue is a multifactorial process. Not all causes are known and the underlying mechanisms leading to fatigue are often poorly understood. It remains to be clarified whether multiple causes act through common or different mechanisms and whether there is a possible additivity of different causes and mechanisms.

In this chapter we will review the identifiable factors leading to fatigue in cancer patients and try to define the underlying mechanisms as well as the therapeutic options that may be derived from them.

Fatigue associated with type, stage and sites of cancer

Fatigue observed in cancer patients appears to be related to disease stage and site. It is often difficult when analysing the causes of fatigue in a patient to dis-

Address for correspondence: M. Marty, Direction de la Recherche Thérapeutique, Institut Gustave Roussy, 39, rue Camille Desmoulins, 94805 Villejuif, France. Tel.: +33-1-42114672, fax: +33-1-42115322, e-mail: marty@igr.fr

tinguish between early or late consequences of therapy and the progression of the disease itself.

Common mechanisms responsible for fatigue in patients with advanced cancer

Whatever the type of primary tumor, common mechanisms related to disease extent and tumor burden can be identified

Dyspnoea is a devastating symptom in patients with advanced cancer and is closely correlated with fatigue, being observed in 50% of patients with very advanced cancer [1,2]. Numerous causes account for dyspnoea including lung and pleural involvement, airway obstruction, anaemia and anxiety [3]. Dyspnoea is responsible for increased energy requirement [4], decrease in saturated haemoglobin, muscle loss and acidosis. All of these can contribute to fatigue.

Denutrition is a frequent finding in patients with advanced cancer. It culminates in the cancer cachexia syndrome, which is clinically characterized by anorexia, weight loss, weakness, fatigue, poor performance status, muscle waste, and impaired immune function; all these symptoms are unresolved by forced caloric intake [5-7]. A number of cytokines, including tumor necrosis factor-alpha, interleukins 1 and 6, IFN-gamma, leukaemia inhibitory factor, and ciliary neurotrophic factor have been proposed as mediators of the cachectic process. High serum levels of some of these cytokines, including IL-1, IL-6 and TNF, are present in advanced-stage cancer patients suffering from denutrition [8]. TNF has been shown to inhibit serum and insulin-like growth factor-I stimulated protein synthesis and to activate protein turnover in the muscles [9,10]; IL-6 induces proteolysis and muscle atrophy [11]. Anti-cytokine and anti-cytokine-receptor therapy inhibits experimental cancer cachexia [12].

Anaemia is recognised as one of the most frequent causes of fatigue in cancer patients [13], to the extent that a Functional Assessment of Cancer Therapy-Anaemia (FACT-An) has been designed and validated. Haemoglobin levels below 11 g% can be responsible for fatigue [14]; fatigue increases with decreasing haematocrit and haemoglobin levels. The beneficial effects of transfusions, correction of iron and vitamin deficiency [15], and corrective or preventive recombinant erythropoietin administration are well documented [16]. Anaemia and its management are discussed by D. Bron, L. Itri and F. Mercuriali in this volume.

Endocrine disorders and metabolic abnormalities

Various hormonal deficiencies can be responsible for fatigue, including hypothyroidism, hypoaldosteronism, Addison's syndrome, and sex hormone deficiency. Such deficiencies are encountered in some advanced cancers and are often due to involvement of the secreting gland by the primary tumour or by metastasis. Furthermore, hormonal deficiencies and/or decreased response of target tissues to hormones have been reported in cachectic patients. Inappropriate and often ectopic secretion of hormones by tumours may also cause fatigue. Hypersecretion of parathyroid hormone [17], adrenal cortex hormones [18], and antidiuretic hormone - acting through its metabolic consequences - are among the most frequently reported hormonal causes of fatigue in patients with cancer.

Paraneoplastic syndromes are generally associated with fatigue. The underlying mechanism(s) are more complex, involving ectopic hormonal secretion [19], autoimmune manifestations such as myositis and/or myasthenia, as well as fluid and metabolic imbalances as induced by SIADH.

Metabolic abnormalities are frequent in advanced cancer. The causes are numerous, involving reduced intake, increased loss through diarrhoea and emesis, and hypercalcaemia in relation to bone metastasis. All can be responsible for fatigue.

Depression, anxiety and sleep disturbances

These conditions are observed in 30% to 80% of cancer patients depending on disease stage, effectiveness and side effects of therapy, and type and effectiveness of psychological support. All may lead to fatigue. They are treated in this volume by S. Dolbeault and A. Glaus.

Fatigue associated with cancer therapy

It has been established for many therapeutic approaches that the treatment of cancer is responsible for fatigue.

Surgery

Fatigue has been repeatedly reported following surgery. Its incidence and severity depend on the type of anaesthesia, the invasiveness of the surgical procedure [20], and early aggressive perioperative care [21]. Covariates for surgery-induced fatigue are pain and its perioperative management, blood loss, postoperative nutrition and early mobilisation. Some aspects of the metabolic changes (increase in blood glucose and decrease in serum albumin) and acute-phase responses (secretion of IL-6 and increase in C-reactive protein) are attenuated following less invasive procedures, consistent with a reduction in tissue trauma [22].

Long-term complications of surgery including malabsorption in extensive intestinal resections and chronic respiratory failure following thoracic surgery contribute to long-lasting fatigue.

Radiotherapy

Fatigue is reported in up to 80% of patients receiving radiation therapy [23-25]. The incidence and severity of fatigue depend on the irradiated volume and involved organs. Possible covariates are radiation-induced pain and dysphagia, anxiety, nutritional status and anaemia. Fatigue usually appears during the second half of radiotherapy, reaches its maximum between completion and four weeks following completion of radiotherapy, and may persist as long as nine months [26]. Few, if any, studies have addressed the influence of the energy and/or fractionation used, or the correlation with the well-known immune depression induced by radiation therapy.

Anticancer agents

Fatigue is reported in patients receiving palliative or curative drug therapy [27-29]. Different and possibly combined patterns of fatigue have been described:

1 *Acute and rapidly reversible fatigue following discontinuous administration of drug therapy:* The causality of the agent(s) used is likely in this setting, particularly in the first administration(s) since anaemia, denutrition, metabolic and other cumulative side effects are not observed during the first administration(s). Possible covariates are anxiety, sleep disturbance and drug-induced emesis. Situations where single agents are used in normal subjects (including healthy volunteers) such as PBPC donors primed with haemopoietic growth factors [30,31] are the most informative because there are no disease-related causes: 15-25% of such normal subjects experience fatigue following a single short course of G-CSF. Reversible fatigue has been reported more frequently with some agents (Table 1). While the degree of drug-induced fatigue is far from being precisely defined and may very well depend on investigator awareness, it is likely that some of these agents induce fatigue quite frequently. This is well established for cytokines and/or interferon given for short periods [32,33]. Interestingly, the effects on the endogenous production of cytokines (IL-1-beta, IL-6, IFN-gamma, TNF-alpha and TNF-beta) are quite variable, with decreases in these markers following interferon-beta therapy [34] and increases following treatment with interferon-alpha and other cytokines [35]. Hormonal alterations due to interferon, in particular hypothyroidism, are frequent and may contribute to fatigue, although they do not appear early during interferon therapy [36]. Therapy with humanised monoclonal antibodies may also lead to fatigue, particularly following the first administration.

2 *Progressive and cumulative fatigue during drug therapy:* Here again convincing arguments for the causality of the agents used are found in subjects given adjuvant therapy or without evidence of progression. One specific situation is the use of sex hormone deprivation therapy [37-40]: metabolic effects on bone and muscles (muscle atrophy) as well as sleep disturbances (related in particular to hot flashes) and depression all contribute to the fatigue observed in 15-30% of such patients. Fatigue has been convincingly reported in patients receiving prolonged interferon therapy (for neoplastic or non-neoplastic disease) and in patients receiving prolonged chemotherapy or repeated cycles of chemotherapy. Again, the most valid interpretations are

Table 1. Anticancer agents associated with fatigue

Agent	Possible causes	Comments
Androgen deprivation therapy	Decreased testosterone levels	
Amifostine		Low daily dose
Aromatase inhibitor (specific)	Decreased oestradiol levels	
Bexarotene		
Cisplatinum	Anaemia, hypomagnesaemia	
Irinotecan		
Corticosteroids	Muscle atrophy	
Docetaxel	Cumulative? Appears after four cycles while no cumulative neutropenia is observed	Dose related
Gemcitabine		
GARFT inhibitors	Anaemia	
HuMAb	Infusion related	Marked during first infusion
Interferons	Associated with depression	Dose related
Radiotherapy	Dose and field dependent	
Raltitrexed	Flu-like syndrome	
rhGM-CSF		
rhG-CSF		15-25% in normal subjects
Thalidomide		
Vinorelbine		2-3 days' duration

obtained in patients with no evidence of disease, i.e., in the adjuvant setting. The mechanisms, which vary widely depending on the type of agent and the dosage, include the following: anaemia; metabolic disorders such as phosphate and magnesium depletion, often related to tubular damage as observed with ifosfamide [41] and cisplatin [42]; fluid imbalance due to severe emesis, drug-induced diarrhoea and drug-induced inappropriate ADH secretion as observed with vinca alkaloids and cyclophosphamide; neurotoxicity with amyotrophy as can be induced by vinca alkaloids and organoplatinum compounds; muscle wasting as observed during septic shock but also TNF therapy (isolated limb infusion) and in experimental models [43]; weight changes, anxiety and depression. Little is known about specific biological abnormalities associated with such treatments nor about possible specific prevention and/or correction of fatigue apart from correction of the metabolic abnormalities observed.

3 *Persisting fatigue in patients who have completed drug therapy and are free of disease:* As mentioned earlier, fatigue lasting for weeks or months is reported in 30% of such patients: no specific biological abnormalities other than drug-related menopausal status and some degree of immunosuppression have been consistently reported. Anxiety and depression are reported in 30-40% of such patients.

4 *General conclusions:* Fatigue is usually related to the dosage of anticancer agents; when combination drug therapy is employed, the incidence and severity of fatigue usually increase. Little is known about the different degrees of fatigue in relation to type of combination regimen, dose, schedule and duration of therapy as independent prognosticators of fatigue (with adjustment for known causes of fatigue such as anaemia). Now that correction of anaemia can be achieved with erythropoietin, it would be interesting to study patients randomised to different combinations for the same type of cancer and with similar haematocrit and/or haemoglobin levels.

Biological abnormalities associated with fatigue

A number of biological abnormalities are associated with fatigue. The fact that they are observed in cancer patients suffering from either disease- or treatment-related fatigue and in fatigue syndromes unrelated to cancer strengthens their causal relationship to fatigue and indicates possible clues with regard to intervention. They are summarised in Table 2.

Immunological abnormalities have repeatedly been quoted as forming the basis of the chronic fatigue syndrome and as being involved in fatigue observed in various diseases including cancer. Few abnormalities have been consistently reported [44]. The most noticeable is low-level activation of the immune system and specifically of the effectors involved in the acute-phase reactions of the inflammatory response such as interleukin-1-beta, interleukin-1 receptor antagonist, soluble interleukin-1 receptor type II, interleukin-6 and tumour necrosis factor [8,22,45-51]. The modest differences indicate that cytokine deregulation is not a singular or dominant factor in the pathogenesis of fatigue although administration of cytokines is usually responsible for a high degree of fatigue, and suggest that anticytokine therapy can reduce fatigue in experimental models.

Table 2. Biological abnormalities associated with fatigue

Abnormality	Biology	Covariates
Low-level activation of the immune system	Increased secretion of interleukin-1 receptor antagonist	
Decreased gonadotropin	Decreased oestrogens	Hot flashes, insomnia
Hypogonadism	Low oestrogens or androgens	
Anaemia	>2 g loss of Hb	
Adrenal insufficiency		Radiotherapy, corticosteroids, aminoglutethimide
Increased TNF-α	Muscle waste	
Increased IL-1		
Increased IL-6		
Phosphate depletion	Abnormal oxidative metabolism	

Hormonal deficiency is one of the most consistent findings. Reduced levels of sex hormones is one of the most frequent abnormalities, in particular in female cancers, and may be related to age, therapeutic suppression of oestrogen production, and lack of hormone replacement therapy. Similar abnormalities are observed in men with reduced levels of testosterone. Correction of the hormonal deficiency has been shown to resolve fatigue (see chapter by S. Pecorelli and L. Fallo in this volume). Causes of fatigue associated with hypogonadism are complex and include hot flashes and sleep disturbance, depression, reduced muscle mass, etc. [24,37,52]. Growth hormone deficiency is well documented in children who have been treated for cancer [53], and the beneficial effects of replacement therapy are established in this setting [54]. In view of the multiple causes of somatotrophin deficiency in adult patients with cancer [55] and the beneficial effects of somatotrophin administration on increased catabolism, fatigue, and muscular mass, surprisingly few studies have been dedicated to growth hormone deficiency and its consequences in patients with cancer. Similarly, while multiple causes of adrenal insufficiency (including involvement of subrenal glands by the tumour, long-term use of glucocorticoids, radiation therapy involving the area, long-term inhibition of P450) are known, few studies have been dedicated to it.

Ion abnormalities are also frequent in cancer patients. It has been hypothe-sised that abnormal ion exchange underlies the fatigue syndrome [56,57]. The involved ions – calcium, phosphorus, magnesium and potassium – are intracellu-lar ones that may not always be properly assessed by measurement of their lev-els in blood [57-60]. Chronic diarrhoea is responsible for dehydration and metabolic abnormalities (potassium, calcium and phosphate depletion) causing fatigue. Hyper- and hypocalcaemia are frequent and should be corrected when-ever found.

Anaemia is one of the prominent causes of fatigue in cancer patients and should be corrected whenever it is encountered.

Some directions for the treatment of fatigue in cancer patients

Treating fatigue in cancer patients is a two-step process. Firstly, known abnor-malities responsible for fatigue should be corrected: all possible known causes of fatigue should be identified and corrected and the fatigue should subsequently be reassessed. This step encompasses pain control, alleviation of anxiety and depression, correction of metabolic abnormalities, nutritional support, hormone replacement therapy when not contraindicated, and correction of anaemia [14, 37,61-63]. No studies on the comprehensive, non-specific management of fatigue in cancer have been reported. It is likely that – as observed in patients with AIDS – a substantial level of fatigue will still be observed in patients with ad-vanced cancer. Secondly, specific approaches to resolving fatigue in cancer pa-tients are based on hormonal manipulation and cytokine manipulation.

Hormonal manipulation. The use of high-dose progestins (megestrol acetate: 250 mg then 160 mg/d) [64] has been extensively studied in patients with AIDS and patients with cancer. The rationales for the use of high-dose progestins are the effects on anorexia and muscle loss, but also systemic responses to cytokines [8]. They also have a rapid effect on weight: maximum weight gain is normally achieved within eight weeks; the weight gain is, unfortunately, mainly due to an increase in fat mass and partly to oedema [65]. Recent studies with lower doses of megestrol acetate (160 mg/d) show a fast (<10 days) positive effect on fatigue. However, it is unlikely that altering the dose and schedule of pro-gestins can improve these results.

Cytokine manipulation. The postulated role of the cytokines IL-1, IL-6 and TNF-alpha on the incidence and severity of fatigue has led investigators to study possible antagonists of such effectors. It is possible to antagonise IL-6 ac-tivation using anti-IL-6 receptor humanised antibody as currently studied in Castleman's disease [66]; no data are available on fatigue syndromes, nor on the side effects of long-term administration of such antibodies. Inhibitors such as suramin have shown positive effects in experimental preclinical models of cachexia [12]. Other approaches involve inhibition of TNF-alpha [12], but no adequate preclinical studies have yet been conducted. It is likely that these therapeutic approaches will be studied in the coming years.

Conclusion

At present, the availability of validated assessment tools for fatigue and a better understanding of the causes and covariates of fatigue in cancer patients allow for adequate recognition of the symptom and its severity as well as identification of the underlying causes and their correction. The efficiency of such preventive and corrective measures has not yet been accurately defined, so it is not known whether further specific therapeutic tools are needed. Hormonal manipulation on the one hand and manipulation of the early inflammatory cytokine response on the other are paths which are currently being explored.

References

1   Bruera E, Schmitz B, Pither J, Neumann CM, Hanson J. The frequency and correlates of dyspnea. J Pain Symptom Manage 2000; 19: 357-62
2   Okuyama T, Akechi T, Kugaya A, et al. Factors correlated with fatigue in disease-free breast cancer patients: application of the Cancer Fatigue Scale. Support Care Cancer 2000; 8: 215-22
3   Tomiska M, Dastych M, Dolezalova J, Vorlicek J. Dyspnea in cancer patients. Etiology, resource utilization, and survival-implications in a managed care world. Cancer 1996; 78: 1314-9
4   Skeletal muscle dysfunction in chronic obstructive pulmonary disease. A statement of the American Thoracic Society and European Respiratory Society. Am J Respir Crit Care Med 1999; 159: S1-40
5   Frost RA, Lang CH, Gelato MC. Effects of cachexia due to cancer on whole body and skeletal muscle protein turnover. Cancer 1998; 82: 42-8.
6   Ling PR, Schwartz JH, Bistrian BR. Muscle hypercatabolism during cancer cachexia is not reversed by the glucocorticoid receptor antagonist RU38486. Cancer Lett 1996; 99: 7-14
7   Strang P. The cancer cachexia syndrome. Semin Oncol 1997; 24: 277-87
8   Strassmann G, Kambayashi T. Cytokine activity in cancer-related anorexia/cachexia: role of megestrol acetate and medroxyprogesterone acetate. Semin Oncol 1998; 25: 45-52
9   Sen CK, Khanna S, Reznick AZ, Roy S, Packer L. Transient exposure of human myoblasts to tumor necrosis factor-alpha inhibits serum and insulin-like growth factor-I stimulated protein synthesis. Endocrinology 1997; 138: 4153-9
10 Tisdale MJ, McDevitt TM, Todorcv PT, Cariuk P. TNF activates protein turnover in skeletal muscle of tumor-bearing animals (Meeting abstract). Proc Annu Meet Am Assoc Cancer Res 1997; 38: A785
11 Anker SD, Ponikowski PP, Clark AL, et al. Interleukin 6 receptor antibody inhibits muscle atrophy and modulates proteolytic systems in interleukin 6 transgenic mice. J Clin Invest 1996; 97: 244-9
12 Inui A. Inhibition of experimental cancer cachexia by anti-cytokine and anti-cytokine-receptor therapy. Cytokines Mol Ther 1995; 1: 107-13
13 Glaus A, Muller S. Hemoglobin and fatigue in cancer patients: inseparable twins? (in German). Schweiz Med Wochenschr 2000; 130: 471-7
14 Itri LM. Optimal hemoglobin levels for cancer patients. Semin Oncol 2000; 27: 12-5
15 Waltzman R, Pezzulli S, Anderson K, et al. Clinical guidelines for the treatment of cancer-related anemia. Pharmacotherapy 1998; 18: 156-69
16 Ludwig H. Epoetin in cancer-related anaemia. Nephrol Dial Transplant 1999; 14 (suppl 2): 85-92

17 Sato S, Yokoyama A, Ohtsuka T, et al. A case of primary hyperparathyroidism that had been treated under a diagnosis of depression for 10 years. Psychiatry Clin Neurosci 1995; 49: 147-9

18 Abasiyanik A, Oran B, Kaymakci A, Yasar C, Caliskan U, Erkul I. Cushing's syndrome due to small cell lung cancer with ectopic production of adrenocorticotropic and parathyroid hormone. Nippon Ronen Igakkai Zasshi 1997; 34: 215-20

19 Jones TH, Wadler S, Hupart KH. Ganglioneuroblastoma of the thymus: an adult case with the syndrome of inappropriate secretion of antidiuretic hormone. Hum Pathol 1996; 27: 506-9

20 Irvine DM, Vincent L, Graydon JE, Bubela N. Postoperative pain and fatigue after laparoscopic or conventional colorectal resections. A prospective randomized trial. Surg Endosc 1998; 12: 1131-6

21 Jakeways MS, Mitchell V, Hashim IA, et al. Recovery after laparoscopic colonic surgery with epidural analgesia, and early oral nutrition and mobilisation. Lancet 1995; 345: 763-4

22 Gaston-Johansson F, Fall-Dickson JM, Bakos AB, Kennedy MJ. Metabolic and inflammatory responses after open or laparoscopic cholecystectomy. Br J Surg 1994; 81: 127-31

23 Bardram L, Funch-Jensen P, Jensen P, Crawford ME, Kehlet H. Frequency and correlates of fatigue in lung cancer patients receiving radiation therapy: implications for management. J Pain Symptom Manage 1996; 11: 370-7

24 Stone P, Hardy J, Broadley K, Tookman AJ, Kurowska A, A'Hern R. Prospective study of fatigue in localized prostate cancer patients undergoing radiotherapy. Radiat Oncol Investig 1997: 178-85

25 Berger AM. Fatigue in women with breast cancer receiving radiation therapy. Cancer Nurs 1998; 21: 127-35

26 Dreisbach AW, Hendrickson T, Beezhold D, Riesenberg LA, Sklar AH. Fatigue and radiotherapy: (B) experience in patients 9 months following treatment. Br J Cancer 1998; 78: 907-12

27 Kaasa S, Loge JH, Knobel H, Jordhoy MS, Brenne E. Fatigue patterns observed in patients receiving chemotherapy and radiotherapy. Cancer Invest 2000; 18: 11-9

28 Kramer JA, Curran D, Piccart M, et al. Identification and interpretation of clinical and quality of life prognostic factors for survival and response to treatment in first-line chemotherapy in advanced breast cancer. Eur J Cancer 2000; 36: 1498-506

29 Broeckel JA, Jacobsen PB, Horton J, Balducci L, Lyman GH. Characteristics and correlates of fatigue after adjuvant chemotherapy for breast cancer. J Clin Oncol 1998; 16: 1689-96

30 Murata M, Harada M, Kato S, et al. Peripheral blood stem cell mobilization and apheresis: analysis of adverse events in 94 normal donors. Bone Marrow Transplant 1999; 24: 1065-71

31 Stroncek DF, Clay ME, Petzoldt ML, et al. Treatment of normal individuals with granulocyte-colony-stimulating factor: donor experiences and the effects on peripheral blood CD34+ cell counts and on the collection of peripheral blood stem cells [see comments]. Transfusion 1996; 36: 601-10

32 Cotler SJ, Wartelle CF, Larson AM, Gretch DR, Jensen DM, Carithers RL Jr. Pretreatment symptoms and dosing regimen predict side-effects of interferon therapy for hepatitis C. J Viral Hepat 2000; 7: 211-7

33 Budman DR, Petroni G, Cooper MR, Schlossman DR, Johnson J, Peterson B. Phase I trial of subcutaneous (SC) interleukin-12 (rHuIL-12) in patients with metastatic renal cell carcinoma (RCC). Proc Annu Meet Am Soc Clin Oncol 1997; 16: A377

34 Rothuizen LE, Buclin T, Spertini F, et al. Influence of interferon beta-1a dose frequency on PBMC cytokine secretion and biological effect markers. J Neuroimmunol 1999; 99: 131-41

35 Jones TH, Wadler S, Hupart KH. Endocrine-mediated mechanisms of fatigue during treatment with interferon-alpha. Semin Oncol 1998; 25 (suppl 1): 54-63

36 Subramanian S, Goker H, Kanji A, Sweeney H. Clinical adrenal insufficiency in patients receiving megestrol therapy. Arch Intern Med 1997; 157: 1008-11

37 Boccardo F. Hormone therapy of prostate cancer: Is there a role for antiandrogen monotherapy? Crit Rev Oncol Hematol 2000; 35: 121-32

38 Herr HW, O'Sullivan M. Quality of life of asymptomatic men with nonmetastatic prostate cancer on androgen deprivation therapy. J Urol 2000; 163: 1743-6

39 Stone P, Hardy J, Huddart R, A'Hern R, Richards M. Fatigue in patients with prostate cancer receiving hormone therapy. Eur J Cancer 2000; 36: 1134-41

40 Clemett D, Lamb HM. Exemestane: a review of its use in postmenopausal women with advanced breast cancer. Drugs 2000; 59: 1279-96

41 Ida T, Kaneko S. Evaluating a critically ill patient with metabolic acidosis: the ifosfamide paradigm. Nephrol Dial Transplant 1999; 14: 226-30

42 Lehrich RW, Moll S, Luft FC. Effect of low-dose prophylactic dopamine on high-dose cisplatin-induced electrolyte wasting, ototoxicity, and epidermal growth factor excretion: a randomized, placebo-controlled, double-blind trial. J Clin Oncol 1995; 13: 1231-7

43 Tsujinaka T, Fujita J, Ebisui C, et al. Mechanisms of host wasting induced by administration of cytokines in rats. Am J Physiol 1997; 272: E333-9

44 Vollmer-Conna U, Lloyd A, Hickie I, Wakefield D. Chronic fatigue syndrome: an immunological perspective. Aust NZ J Psychiatry 1998; 32: 523-7

45 Cannon JG, Angel JB, Ball RW, Abad LW, Fagioli L, Komaroff AL. Acute phase responses and cytokine secretion in chronic fatigue syndrome. J Clin Immunol 1999; 19: 414-21

46 MacDonald KL, Osterholm MT, LeDell KH, et al. A case-control study to assess possible triggers and cofactors in chronic fatigue syndrome. Am J Med 1996; 100: 548-54

47 Nyberg P, Wikman AL, Nennesmo I, Lundberg I. Increased expression of interleukin 1-alpha and MHC class I in muscle tissue of patients with chronic, inactive polymyositis and dermatomyositis. J Rheumatol 2000; 27: 940-8

48 Monga U, Jaweed M, Kerrigan AJ, et al. Elevated levels of tumor necrosis factor alpha in postdialysis fatigue. Int J Artif Organs 1998; 21: 83-6

49 Hasselgren PO, Fischer JE. Sepsis: stimulation of energy-dependent protein breakdown resulting in protein loss in skeletal muscle. World J Surg 1998; 22: 203-8

50 Moss RB, Mercandetti A, Vojdani A. TNF-alpha and chronic fatigue syndrome. J Clin Immunol 1999; 19: 314-6

51 Ostrowski K, Rohde T, Asp S, Schjerling P, Pedersen BK. Pro- and anti-inflammatory cytokine balance in strenuous exercise in humans. J Physiol (Lond) 1999; 515: 287-91

52 Dionne IJ, Kinaman KA, Poehlman ET. Sarcopenia and muscle function during menopause and hormone-replacement therapy. J Nutr Health Aging 2000; 4: 156-61

53 Brook CG. Which children should receive growth hormone treatment. Reserve it for the GH deficient. Arch Dis Child 2000; 83: 176-8

54 Moshang T Jr. Use of growth hormone in children surviving cancer. Med Pediatr Oncol 1998; 31: 170-2

55 Wallymahmed ME, Foy P, MacFarlane IA. The quality of life of adults with growth hormone deficiency: comparison with diabetic patients and control subjects. Clin Endocrinol (Oxf) 1999; 51: 333-8

56 Chaudhuri A, Watson WS, Pearn J, Behan PO. The symptoms of chronic fatigue syndrome are related to abnormal ion channel function. Med Hypotheses 2000; 54: 59-63

57 Baker AJ, Carson PJ, Miller RG, Weiner MW. Metabolic and nonmetabolic components of fatigue monitored with 31P-NMR. Muscle Nerve 1994; 17: 1002-9

58 Durlach J, Bac P, Durlach V, Bara M, Guiet-Bara A. Neurotic, neuromuscular and autonomic nervous form of magnesium imbalance. Magnes Res 1997; 10: 169-95

59 De Lorenzo F, Hargreaves J, Kakkar VV. Phosphate diabetes in patients with chronic fatigue syndrome. Postgrad Med J 1998; 74: 229-32

60 Yu-Yahiro JA. Electrolytes and their relationship to normal and abnormal muscle function. Orthop Nurs 1994; 13: 38-40

61 Cella D, Bron D. The effect of epoetin alfa on quality of life in anemic cancer patients. Cancer Pract 1999; 7: 177-82

62 Hickok JT, Morrow GR, McDonald S, Bellg AJ. Nutritional aspects of cancer-related fatigue. J Am Diet Assoc 1997; 97: 650-4

63 Land JM, Kemp GJ, Taylor DJ, Standing SJ, Radda GK, Rajagopalan B. Oral phosphate supplements reverse skeletal muscle abnormalities in a case of chronic fatigue with idiopathic renal hypophosphatemia. Neuromuscul Disord 1993; 3: 223-5

64 Watanabe S, Pituskin E, Calder K, Neumann C, Bruera E. Effectiveness of megestrol acetate in patients with advanced cancer: a randomized, double-blind, crossover study. Cancer Prev Control 1998; 2: 74-8

65 Anker SD, Rauchhaus M. The effect of megestrol acetate on anorexia, weight loss and cachexia in cancer and AIDS patients (review). Anticancer Res 1997; 17: 657-62

66 Nielsen SE, Zeuthen J, Lund B, Persson B, Alenfall J, Hansen HH. Improvement in Castleman's disease by humanized anti-interleukin-6 receptor antibody therapy. Blood 2000; 95: 56-61

ESO Scientific Updates, Vol. 5
Fatigue and Cancer
M. Marty and S. Pecorelli, editors
© 2001 Elsevier Science B.V. All rights reserved

Biological Basis of Cancer-Related Anaemia

Dominique Bron

Institut Jules Bordet, Brussels, Belgium

Introduction

Anaemia, which occurs in more than 50% of cancer patients, represents a major cause of fatigue in this population. Several factors may cause anaemia; these are either directly related to the tumour (blood loss, haemolysis, bone marrow infiltration, hypersplenism, nutrient deficiencies) or result from treatment (chemotherapy or radiation). In a considerable number of patients, however, no causes other that the malignant disease itself can be implicated [1].

The impact of anaemia on physical and cognitive capacities varies considerably among individuals. However, a linear correlation between haemoglobin levels and relevant quality of life parameters has been reported in several studies and indicates the importance of adequate treatment of anaemia and maintenance of an optimal haemogloblin level.

This chapter deals with normal haematopoiesis as well as the pathophysiology and treatment of cancer-related anaemia.

Haematopoiesis and erythropoiesis

Haematopoiesis is constantly required because of normal turnover in blood cell populations. Erythropoiesis is part of the process of haematopoiesis, producing more than 10^{11} erythrocytes daily.

Erythropoiesis is finely regulated to maintain the normal number of circulating blood erythrocytes. The major stages of differentiation are shown in Figure 1. Normal pluripotent haematopoietic stem cells maintain adequate differentiated haematopoietic cell production. The normal pluripotent stem cell has the ability to self-replicate but also to differentiate into committed progenitors under the complex regulation of the bone marrow microenvironment and haematopoietic growth factors.

Address for correspondence: D. Bron, Institut Jules Bordet, 1 rue Héger-Bordet, 1000 Brussels, Belgium. Tel.: +32-2-5413232, fax: +32-2-5440257, e-mail: dbron@ulb.ac.be

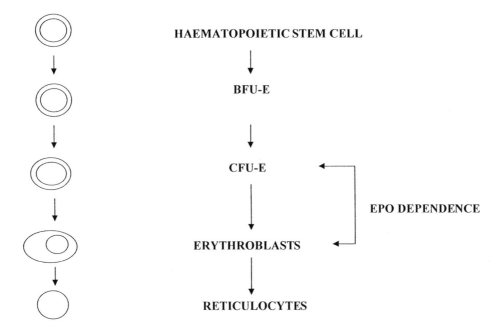

Fig. 1. Major stages of erythropoiesis and EPO dependence

The most immature stage of committed erythroid progenitors is the burst forming unit erythroid (BFU-E). Human BFU-E requires 14 days or more to develop into clusters of mature erythroblasts. The next major stage of erythroid progenitor cell development is the colony forming unit erythroid (CFU-E). Human CFU-E requires only seven days to develop into single clusters of eight to 64 mature erythroblasts. The descendant cells of the CFU-E are erythroid "precursors cells". The last stage, the orthochromatic erythroblasts, do not divide but they enucleate, forming the reticulocyte.

Essential nutrients such as iron, folate and vitamin B12 are required for the normal differentiation and proliferation of erythroid progenitor cells. Among the various growth factors influencing erythroid progenitor cell proliferation, erythropoietin (EPO) is the most important. There is no erythropoiesis in the absence of EPO. C-kit ligand (stem cell factor) is a non-specific growth factor acting at an early stage of erythropoiesis, but the fine regulation of erythropoiesis is not yet fully understood.

Production of erythropoietin

Erythropoietin (EPO) is a glycoprotein hormone produced mainly by renal cortical cells and also by hepatocytes. It is produced in response to hypoxia generally related to the number of circulating erythrocytes. Under normal conditions any loss of erythrocytes (bleeding, haemolysis) decreases delivery of oxygen to the tissue. The hypoxia is sensed by an intracellular molecule that interacts with an enhancer element of the EPO gene, inducing transcription of the gene and thereby leading to EPO secretion into the plasma. Arriving in the bone marrow, EPO binds to specific cell-surface receptors on CFU-E and erythroid precursors. Because of the small number of receptors, these cells require a high concentration of EPO.

In healthy individuals a linear decrease in haemoglobin level is accompanied by an exponential increase in plasma EPO levels. The increase in EPO production is achieved by recruitment of more renal tubular interstitial cells, whereas liver cells are able to secrete more EPO.

Mechanism of action of EPO

EPO binds to receptors on erythroid precursors, prevents apoptosis and stimulates proliferation and differentiation into reticulocytes. Following cell maturation, the precursors have a reduced capacity for proliferation and acquire more receptors. In hyperoxic situations or kidney diseases the production of EPO falls and EPO-dependent cells undergo apoptosis leading to anaemia. *In vitro* the effect of EPO starts after 2 to 24 hours. In some conditions including cancer the production of EPO in response to the level of anaemia is not optimal and in such cases administration of recombinant human erythropoietin (rHuEPO) might be useful.

Anaemia in cancer patients

More than 50% of cancer patients will become anaemic during the course of their disease and many of them will require red blood cell transfusions. The incidence of anaemia depends on several factors including the type of malignancy, diseage stage and duration, and the intensity of treatment (chemotherapy or radiation).

Anaemia is a common feature in haematological malignancies and in solid tumours with bone metastases. In such situations bone marrow replacement is the major cause of anaemia. Metastases destroy progenitor cells and damage bone marrow stromal cells, thus impairing growth factor production. Some tumours produce cytokines with myelosuppressive effects (e.g. TNF and IFN-γ) [2]. Other tumours, such as breast and prostate cancer, induce fibrotic reactions that disrupt the marrow environment.

Solid tumours such as lung cancer or ovarian cancer, which are often treated with platinum derivatives, are reported to have the highest rates of transfusion requirement (50-100% depending on age of the patient, intensity of chemotherapy, and baseline haemoglobin level). In fact, these platinum-derived drugs are known to affect EPO production due to renal toxicity [3-5]. Other cyto-toxic drugs may cause transient or prolonged anaemia through different mecha-nisms including stem cell damage, blockage of haematopoietic factors, myelo-dysplasia, microangiopathic anaemia, and immune-mediated haematopoietic cell destruction [6].

Leukaemias, lymphomas, myelodysplastic syndromes and multiple myelo-ma are certainly the most frequent cancer types associated with anaemia. The mechanism of anaemia is multifactorial in these diseases and comprises bone marrow involvement, stromal cell damage, amyloid deposition, hypersplenism, coagulation disorders with bleeding, autoimmune haemolysis, haematophago-cytosis as well as chemotherapy, radiotherapy, immunotherapy and infectious complications.

Other factors such as surgical resection, nutritional deficiencies (iron, folic acid), drug nephrotoxicity, endocrine disorders or simply reduced marrow re-serve due to aging also contribute to anaemia.

Cancer-related anaemia

However, in some cancer patients with anaemia none of these causes are evident and the anaemia is thus cancer-related, i.e., primarily due to the presence of malignant cells. The haematological and biological characteristics of cancer-related anaemia (CRA) are very similar to those observed in chronic inflamma-tory diseases, i.e., a low reticulocyte count, low serum iron level, low transferrin saturation, elevated ferritin level and normocytic red blood cells [7].

Recent studies have demonstrated that CRA results from the activation of the immune and inflammatory systems by the malignancy with increased levels of interferons (IFN), tumour-necrosis factor (TNF) and interleukin-1 (IL-1) [8]. The concentration of IFN-γ, as evidenced by an increase in neopterin level, re-flects the link between macrophage activation and anaemia in these patients [9]. TNF might also be increased but this depends on the type of malignancy. There is evidence from in vivo treatment with TNF that chronic exposure to TNF induces anaemia [10,11]. The level of IL-1 has also been shown to be ele-vated and directly related to the degree of anaemia. All these cytokines are known to induce anaemia through a myelosuppressive mechanism.

Besides the decreased rate of red blood cell production in CRA, shortened red cell survival, impaired iron utilisation and inadequate EPO production have been demonstrated (Table 1) [12]. Red blood cells survive 120 days in healthy subjects, while in patients with chronic diseases including cancer they usually survive 60-90 days. This shortened cell survival is correlated with the level of IL-1 in rheumatoid arthritis and the same mechanism could be implicated in CRA. TNF is known to induce dyserythropoiesis and reduced life span of red cells.

The iron metabolism has been studied in various types of malignant disease. Patients with chronic lymphocytic leukaemia, multiple myeloma, malignant

Table 1. Mechanisms involved in cancer-related anaemia

- Inhibition of erythropoiesis (TNF, IFN-γ, IL-1, IL-6)
- Shortened red blood cell survival (60-90 instead of 120 days)
- Impaired iron utilisation
- Inadequate EPO production

---

lymphoma and solid tumours proved to have reduced iron levels and transferrin saturation despite normal ferritin levels. By contrast, in myelodysplastic syndrome and chronic myeloproliferative diseases normal iron levels and transferrin saturation were observed. When a patient is successfully treated with rHu-EPO the serum ferritin level decreases in the early phase of treatment and is predictive of response to rHuEPO, suggesting that high doses of rHuEPO can overcome the impairment of iron mobilisation.

Inflammatory cytokines such as TNF, IL-1 and IFN are known to inhibit erythropoiesis *in vivo*. The inhibitory effect of IL-1 requires the presence of T lymphocytes and is mediated by IFN-γ, whereas TNF requires the presence of marrow stroma. Again, rHuEPO administration can overcome the suppressive effect of these cytokines on erythroid progenitor cells.

In CRA erythroid progenitor cells respond normally to EPO but the EPO production is often not optimal for the level of anaemia [14]. To express the best value of EPO, the ratio of observed-to-predicted (O/P) EPO level has been evaluated in various cancer groups. The median O/P ratio in patients with myelodysplasia (MDS) was significantly higher than in the other groups of cancer patients. The lowest O/P ratio was observed in malignant lymphomas, multiple myeloma and solid tumours. In patients with multiple myeloma and creatinine levels above 1.5 mg/dl the O/P ratio was even lower (0.47 versus 0.78). The EPO response may additionally be suppressed by hyperviscosity, which is frequently associated with multiple myeloma.

TNF and IL-1 are cytokines that were shown to inhibit EPO production in hepatoblastoma cell cultures and in isolated perfused rat kidneys. These cytokines are therefore likely to be involved in the reduction of EPO production in lymphoproliferative diseases.

In addition, as mentioned previously, platinum derivatives are nephrotoxic drugs and as such also impair EPO production.

Clinical manifestations of anaemia

The symptoms of anaemia vary among individuals but anaemia is particularly poorly tolerated in patients with impaired cardiac function. Tachycardia, dyspnoea, hypotension and fatigue are the most common features of anaemia, but several other symptoms may be present such as anorexia, mood disturbances, headache, dizziness, reduced cognitive function, and overall diminished well-being [13]. In order to preserve quality of life in cancer patients, the optimum haemoglobin level to be reached is 12 g/dl [15].

In conclusion, anemia is a major complaint in cancer patients, leading to fatigue and impaired quality of life and requiring transfusions in a substantial number of patients. Its causes are not always clear and in the absence of specific treatments the O/P ratio of the EPO level in the serum allows to identify anaemic patients who may benefit from rHuEPO administration.

References

1   Mercadante S, Gebbia V, Marrazzo A, Filosto S. Anaemia in cancer: pathophysiology and treatment. Cancer Treat Rev 2000; 26: 303-11
2   Johnson CS, Cook CA, Furmanski P. In vivo suppression of erythropoiesis (EPO). Exp Hematol 1990; 18: 109-13
3   Canaparo R, Casale F, Muntoni E, et al. Plasma erythropoietin concentrations in patients receiving intensive platinum or nonplatinum chemotherapy. Br J Clin Pharmacol 2000; 50: 146-53
4   Pivot X, Guardiola E, Etienne MC, et al. An analysis of potential factors allowing an individual prediction of cisplatin-induced anaemia. Eur J Cancer 2000; 36: 852-7
5   Wood PA, Hrushesky WJM. Cisplatin-associated anemia: an erythropoietin deficiency syndrome. J Clin Invest 1995; 95: 1650-9
6   Tatcher N. Management of chemotherapy-induced anemia in solid tumors. Semin Oncol 1998; 25 (suppl 7): 23-66
7   Spivak JL. The blood in systemic disorders. Lancet 2000; 355: 1707-12
8   Baraldi-Junkins C, Beckk A, Rothstein G. Hematopoiesis and cytokines. Relevance to cancer and aging. Hematol Oncol Clin N Am 2000; 14: 45-61
9   Means RT. Pathogenesis of the anemia of chronic disease: a cytokine-mediated anemia. Stem Cells 1995; 13: 32-7
10   Broxmeyer HE, Williams DE, Lu L, et al. The suppressive influences of human tumor necrosis factors on bone marrow hematopoietic progenitor cells from normal donors and patients with leukemia: synergism of tumor necrosis factor and interferon-γ. J Immunol 1986; 136: 4487-95
11   Tracey KJ, Wei H, Manogue KR, et al. Cachectin/tumor necrosis factor induces cachexia, anemia and inflammation. J Exp Med 1988; 167: 1211-27
12   Nowrousian MR, Kasper C, Oberhoff C, et al. Pathophysiology of cancer-related anemia. In: Smyth JF, Boogaerts MA, Ehmer BRM, eds. Erythropietin in cancer supportive treatment. New York: Marcel Dekker, 1996; 13-35
13   Cella D, Bron D. The effect of epoietin alfa on quality of life in anemic cancer patients. Cancer Practice 1999; 7: 177-82
14   Ludwig H, Fritz E. Anemia in cancer patients. Prediction of response to EPO. Semin Oncol 1998; 25 (suppl 7): 2-6
15   Itri LM. Optimal hemoglobin levels for cancer patients. Semin Oncol 2000; 27 (suppl 4): 12-5

ESO Scientific Updates, Vol. 5
Fatigue and Cancer
M. Marty and S. Pecorelli, editors

51

Importance of Hormone Replacement Therapy Following Cancer Treatment

Sergio Pecorelli[1,2] and Luca Fallo[1]

1   Department of Obstetrics and Gynaecology, University of Brescia
2   European Institute of Oncology, Milan, Italy

Introduction

Following treatment of cancer, women are often left in an oestrogen-deficient state, and may experience a series of symptoms due to the lack of hormones, either associated with treatment procedures or natural menopause. Moreover, since cancer is being detected at an earlier age and adjuvant treatments can cause ovarian failure, the number of women becoming menopausal at a younger age after cancer treatment is increasing.

Just like women of the general population, women who survived cancer have a risk of developing atherosclerosis, hypertension, cardiovascular diseases and osteoporosis. Hormone replacement therapy (HRT) has been demonstrated to be protective against cardiovascular disease (the leading non-neoplastic cause of death in cancer survivors), and is considered the mainstay of therapy of osteoporosis, which is responsible for the majority of the approximately 1,500,000 fractures each year, a significant cause of mortality in the postmenopausal patient [1-3]. HRT also has the potential to influence brain function, decreasing the relative risk of Alzheimer's disease [4,5]. Hot flushes, sweats, insomnia, depression, increased irritability, fatigue, urogenital atrophy and skin changes have all been experienced by many women who have gone through the menopause: HRT is able to control these symptoms, resulting in significant improvement in quality of life. Thus the issue of HRT in cancer survivors is a very critical one, and for this reason there is great interest in the preservation of the hormonal status of women who have been treated for cancer.

While the issue of administering hormone therapy in most neoplastic diseases has been universally accepted, there is serious concern regarding the use of HRT in the so-called "hormonally sensitive neoplasms". The standard practice

Address for correspondence: S. Pecorelli, Istituto Europeo di Oncologia, Via Ripamonti 435, 20141 Milan, Italy. Tel.: +30-02-57489205, fax: +39-02-57489872,
e-mail: sergio.pecorelli@ieo.it

has been to deny HRT to patients with a previous diagnosis of breast, uterine or ovarian cancer, because doctors have the impression they are pouring fuel on fire. A reappraisal of this practice is essential and must involve a correct analysis of the risks versus benefits of HRT.

The menopause

Menopause is defined as the cessation of the ovarian follicular function resulting in the permanent cessation of menstruation. The median age of onset of menopause is between 50 and 52 years: this means that most women will spend one third of their lives in a condition of oestrogen depletion. In 1990 467 million women were postmenopausal; by 2030, about 76% of postmenopausal women will be living in developing countries, versus 40% in 1990.

Oestrogen deprivation has short- and long-term effects. The early and most commonly reported symptoms in the menopausal transition are typically secondary to vasomotor instability and atrophic changes associated with ovarian failure and subsequent fall in oestrogen levels. The frequency, onset, severity, and duration of symptoms vary between individuals and between ethnic groups. Hot flushes and night sweats affect as many as 75% to 85% of postmenopausal women; the quality of life of women is influenced by psychological and physiological effects such as sleep disturbances, irritability and mood changes including depression.

As women progress through the menopause to the postmenopausal phase, aging and the protracted depletion of oestrogen result in tissue atrophy in several organ systems: it has been reported that as many as one third of women aged 50 years and older experience urogenital problems [6]. Oestrogen deficiency results in atrophy of the urogenital epithelium, vaginal introitus and vulva. The vagina becomes less elastic and the vaginal epithelium becomes thin and less lubricated, especially in response to sexual arousal. These modifications often lead to dyspareunia, vaginitis, pruritus, vaginal stenosis, and atrophic urethral epithelium, with subsequent sexual dysfunction and micturition disorders.

HRT is indicated for the relief of vasomotor symptoms and treatment of urogenital atrophy. Oestrogen has been shown to prevent recurrent urinary tract infections and alleviate symptoms of urgency, urge incontinence, frequency, nycturia and dysuria [7]. However, clinicians should be prepared to discuss with their patients the use of HRT for long-term prophylaxis of osteoporosis, cardiovascular disease, cognitive decline, and Alzheimer's disease. In the postmenopausal phase of life, these long-term consequences of oestrogen loss represent potentially serious threats to the health and longevity of the aging female.

Osteoporosis

Osteoporosis is defined as a disease characterised by low bone mass and microarchitectural deterioration of bone tissue, leading to enhanced bone fragility and therefore to susceptibility to the risk of fractures [8].

Oestrogen deficiency is a dominant pathogenic factor in bone loss: the menopause induces increased bone turnover with a consequent accelerated bone loss especially within 5-6 years, followed by a linear rate that may accelerate again after the age of 75. From 1.5 years before menopause to 1.5 years after menopause, the bone mineral density (BMD) of the spine decreases by 2.5% per year, compared with a premenopausal loss rate of 0.13% per year [9]. Postmenopausal osteoporosis is a major problem in Western countries: an estimated 1.5 million bone fractures occur annually in women because of osteoporosis, the median age at which hip fractures occur being about 80 years. Low bone mineral density is associated with an increased risk of fractures (12-fold for women in the lowest quartile of density) [10].

Several placebo-controlled trials have shown that HRT prevents bone loss in women in the early and late menopause by inhibiting bone cell resorption. HRT is effective in preventing osteoporotic fractures, even when the treatment is initiated later in life, decreasing the risk of hip, spine and wrist fractures by 30-50% [11-17]. After HRT is stopped, bone loss resumes within a year and bone turnover increases to the level of untreated women within 3-6 months: consequently, HRT should be initiated soon after menopause and continued for longer than 10 years, if possible for life [18].

Cardiovascular disease

One in four women dies of coronary heart disease (CHD) and as many as 36% of women aged 55-64 with CHD are disabled by their illness [19,20]. On the basis of epidemiological data there is compelling evidence that HRT reduces the occurrence of CHD, and possibly cerebrovascular disease, by 25-50% compared with no treatment [21,22]. This protective effect of oestrogen is partly due to improvements in the plasma lipid metabolism, lowering cholesterol and LDL cholesterol, inhibiting lipid peroxidation and raising HDL cholesterol [22-25]. Oestrogen may also positively influence carbohydrate metabolism, atheroma formation and cardiovascular haemodynamics, restoring endothelial function, improving cardiac output and arterial flow velocity, and decreasing vascular resistance and systolic and diastolic blood pressure [22]. The only large randomised clinical study on the benefit of HRT in CHD, the HERS study, found no overall effect of HRT on secondary prevention of CHD in postmenopausal women with established CHD over a mean follow-up of four years [26]. The risk was unexpectedly increased in the first four months in the HRT group, followed by a decline to a relative risk of 0.67 in the final two years. Thus, although there is significant evidence that HRT is protective in the primary prevention of CHD, further large-scale studies of HRT in women with established CHD are warranted, especially with different HRT regimens [22,27,28].

The effects of HRT on stroke are uncertain: a recent study found no conclusive evidence that HRT may prevent stroke [29]. Other data demonstrate that HRT is associated with a reduction in stroke mortality as well as stroke incidence [30,31].

Menopause and cognitive function

Oestrogens are known to play a role in many brain processes, through both alpha- and beta-receptors as well as nongenomic pathways [32]. Multiple neuronal functions are influenced by hormones, including those involved in growth, survival and synaptic activity [33-35]. In general, oestrogen has a positive effect on mood and contributes to the sense of well-being, maybe as an effect of the increase in neurotransmitters such as serotonin, acetylcholine, dopamine, noradrenaline, glutamate, gamma-aminobutyric acid and opioid peptides [36]. The long-term action of oestrogen is mediated through both neuroprotective and neurotrophic effects: oestrogen may protect neurons from oxidative, hypoglycaemic and ischaemic injury and may be implicated in the mechanism of neuronal repair through expression of nerve growth factor and stimulation of apolipoprotein E, an injury-response protein that stimulates the regeneration of damaged neurons [37,38]. These effects may be responsible for the mechanism of protection against the development and manifestations of Alzheimer's disease in women who undergo HRT. Epidemiological data demonstrate that a 65-year-old woman has a lifetime risk of developing Alzheimer's disease that approaches one in three and women who take oestrogen after menopause reduce this risk by about 50%, even after only one to two years of HRT [39]. In the prospective study by Tang et al. the rate of increase in the expression of Alzheimer's disease was delayed in oestrogen users: 5% of patients treated with oestrogen postmenopausally developed clinical manifestations of the disease versus 50% of untreated women [40]. There are a number of potential mechanisms by which oestrogen deprivation after the menopause might influence the development of Alzheimer's disease: oestrogens promote neuronal growth and differentiation, influence synaptic plasticity, modulate neurotrophins and neurotransmitter systems, reduce inflammation, oxidation and apoptosis, promote augmentation of cerebral blood flow and metabolism, and reduce amyloid-β protein.

The data on the beneficial effects of oestrogen on the risk of developing Alzheimer's disease are remarkably consistent (RR 0.4-0.6) among case-control and cohort studies [40-46]. The reduction in the risk of Alzheimer's disease appears to be directly proportional to the duration of oestrogen use. Nevertheless, oestrogen has no effect on the treatment of the disease: oestrogen therapy seems to retard the progression but does not seem to influence the final evolution of the disease [47-50].

The observed effects of oestrogen on cognitive function have been inconsistent [51-56]: these results may be due to small sample size or selection biases and to the instruments used to assess the effects [53].

In related studies, oestrogen has been shown to reduce the symptoms of Parkinson's disease and the levodopa requirement in this disease [57,58]. The data on oestrogen and Parkinson's disease are still preliminary. There is, however, sufficient evidence suggestive of beneficial effects to warrant further studies.

Several studies report an increased incidence of vision problems in postmenopausal women [59,60] and some studies suggest that oestrogen use may reduce the incidence of age-related macular degeneration [61].

Breast cancer

The use of HRT in breast cancer survivors is the most sensitive point of the controversy and so much has been written about a possible role of hormones in increasing the risk of cancer of the breast that both medical practitioners and the "patient population" are often thoroughly confused by the issues debated. For many women the benefits of HRT may not compensate for the fear of acquiring breast cancer and living with its effects [62].

Unfortunately, there has never been a large, prospective, double-blind randomised study addressing this issue and thus helping patients and their doctors make a decision. It is therefore necessary to use indirect evidence which can be obtained from past fortuitous exposure of potential or occult breast cancers to endogenous or exogenous oestrogens. Such situations may be a pregnancy coinciding with or subsequent to breast cancer, breast cancer in both previous and current users of oral contraceptives (OC), and breast cancer in postmenopausal women receiving oestrogen replacement therapy (ERT).

Several authors found that the survival of a pregnant patient with breast cancer is comparable to that of a non-pregnant patient of similar age and with similar stage of disease at diagnosis: the additional factor of pregnancy did not confer a worse prognosis, and neither spontaneous nor therapeutic abortion influenced the course of cancer [63,64]. Women who became pregnant after treatment for breast cancer, even within six months, had a survival not different from that of controls [65] or indeed seemed to survive longer [66,67].

A large number of patients diagnosed with breast cancer used OC during the initiation and evolution of their neoplasms. A major study addressing this issue showed there to be no adverse effects of OC use on the outcome of cancer, regardless of the duration of use or latency period [68].

It has been well established in prospective studies that prophylactic oophorectomy does not influence prognosis in premenopausal women with a diagnosis of breast cancer [69]. For this reason it seems irrational that a woman who was 35-40 years old after treatment for breast cancer without oophorectomy cannot use oestrogens when complaining of postmenopausal symptoms 10-15 years later. Many suggest that there is no difference between endogenous and exogenous oestrogens and prohibition of HRT after several years of endogenous hormones does not make sense.

The role played by oestrogen and progesterone in breast cancer remains unclear. The Nachtigall study is the only long-term prospective randomised trial on postmenopausal hormone replacement therapy thus far reported [70]. After 22 years of surveillance, six cases of breast cancer were diagnosed in the 52 women who never received hormone treatment, while there were no cases in the 116 women who did receive HRT; this difference is statistically significant.

Four of the five major meta-analyses in the literature did not report any increased risk in ever versus never users of oestrogen [71-75]. One of these studies found a slightly increased risk if HRT had been used for more than 15 years: this increase was largely based on studies that included premenopausal women and on European studies in which oestradiol (which produces higher circulating levels of oestrogen) was administered. Grady [76] and Colditz [75] reported a significantly higher RR of 1.25 after eight years or longer and 1.23 after ten years or longer of ERT.

A report from the Nurses' Health Study [77] raised alarm among physicians and users: this prospective cohort study found that the risk of breast cancer was increased among women taking oestrogen alone (RR 1.32, CI 1.14-1.54) or oestrogen plus progesterone (RR 1.41, CI 1.15-1.74). Women who had been taking hormones for less than five years were not at risk, while those on HRT for five to nine years had an adjusted RR of 1.46; for ≥10 years of HRT the RR was exactly the same. Despite the large number of patients considered these findings are not definitive and are not free of confounding variables. Detection bias is a major concern: there was a 14% higher prevalence of mammography in HRT users compared to non-users. In the group of current users there were other important characteristics to be taken into account: higher frequency of benign breast disease, lower number of births, and earlier menarche; furthermore, the risk appeared to be limited to women with a body mass index (BMI) between 21 and 23. Although each of these factors alone does not explain the observed outcome, the cumulative effect might. It is also remarkable that the data are not based on the entire patient group but only 71% of them. If we look at the duration of treatment it must be noted that the RR is the same for women treated for five to nine years as for those treated for 15 years: if we consider oestrogen as a carcinogenic agent this is in contrast with toxicology rules. Moreover, the authors found that if HRT is stopped the risk disappears within a short period of time: this is highly unusual and also in contrast with the toxicology rules, which state that the effect of a carcinogen persists for a definite period of time. Lastly, the size of the statistical risk is not outside the range of influence by biases.

In the most recent report from the Nurses' Health Study [78] the authors report a 43% increase in deaths from breast cancer among women who used HRT for 10 years or more. However, the rate of deaths due to breast cancer was higher in the study cohort than in the general population, and this obviously limits the generalisation of the results. Interestingly, this study shows that HRT users with a family history of breast cancer, one of the best known risk factors for this cancer, do not have a greater risk of death from breast cancer than HRT users without this risk factor. The authors state that, "on average, the survival benefits appear to outweigh the risk, but the risks and benefits vary depending on existing risk factors and the duration of hormone use and must be carefully considered for each woman."

The Collaborative Group on Hormonal Factors in Breast Cancer, re-analysing the data on 51,000 women with breast cancer and 108,000 controls (from 51 studies worldwide) reported that ever-use of HRT was associated with an overall increase of 14% in the relative risk of breast cancer, with a 2.3% increase for each year of HRT, which levels off after cessation of HRT [79].

Whereas short-term oestrogen use (less than five years) is not associated with increased breast cancer risk, controversy exists on its long-term use (more than 10 years). The large Swedish epidemiological study of long-term HRT demonstrated a trend towards increasing risk (statistically significant only in women with a BMI lower than 27) with longer duration of use [80]. The excess risk was mainly confined to localised breast cancers: the Collaborative Group and the Iowa Women's Health Study [81] showed that the cancers were less aggressive and the survival was longer in HRT users than in non-users.

To underline the uncertainty of all the conclusions on the link between breast cancer and HRT, a recent prospective cohort study based on a nationally representative cohort followed for 22 years found no statistically significant association between HRT use and subsequent development of breast cancer, including no trend towards a correlation between relative risk and duration of HRT [82].

It has been estimated that the number of breast cancer survivors in the United States may approach 2.5 million. As the effect of oestrogens on breast cancer remains unknown, there are essentially no data and considerable controversy on the effects of HRT following treatment of breast cancer [83]. There are a few uncontrolled studies which addressed this issue: DiSaia et al. [84] reported their experience with 77 breast cancer survivors who had HRT for a median of 59 months after treatment for breast cancer. Forty-nine patients had either stage 0 (6) or stage 1 (43) disease. Seven (9%) patients developed recurrences, while 55/58 node-negative and 10/13 node-positive patients remained without evidence of disease. The authors suggested that hormonal exposure does not cause recurrence as was feared, and their findings do not support the "fuel-on-fire" theory.

In a later re-evaluation [85] DiSaia et al. demonstrated no adverse effect of HRT administered to breast cancer survivors. Forty-one patients from a group of 77 patients who received HRT after breast cancer treatment were matched with 82 patients not receiving HRT. An analysis of survival time and disease-free interval revealed no statistically significant difference between the two groups.

Powles [86], Stoll [87], Wile [88], Eden [89] and Vassilopolou-Sellin [90] showed no evidence of disease progression or recurrence in patients with breast cancer treated with HRT. A recent prospective study of HRT after localised breast cancer indicates that HRT does not seem to increase breast cancer events [91].

Endometrial cancer

Adenocarcinoma of the endometrium has been traditionally considered an "oestrogen-dependent" tumour, and the traditional post-hysterectomy management regimens therefore precluded the use of ERT. In addition, endometrial cancer patients who underwent surgery suffer from considerable vasomotor symptoms as a result of bilateral oophorectomy; many who are several years postmenopausal will also develop these symptoms following surgery, probably because of removal of the androgens produced by the ovarian stroma which are peripherally converted to oestrogens. To date there are no prospective randomised trials utilising ERT or HRT after primary therapy for endometrial cancer and it is therefore necessary to rely on theoretical assumptions and indirect evidence.

In a retrospective review of 221 stage I endometrial cancer patients, 47 receiving oestrogen and 174 controls, the oestrogen-treated group experienced longer disease-free survival after controlling for other risk factors. The prognostic factors (grade, depth of myometrial infiltration, node metastases, peritoneal cytology, hormone receptors) were not statistically different between the two groups. Among the controls there were 26 recurrences and 26 deaths, 16 from cancer and 10 from intercurrent disease. Among the oestrogen-treated women there were one recurrence and one death [92].

A second retrospective study on the use of oral oestrogens confirmed these findings: in this study it is remarkable that five of eight non-oestrogen-treated patients dying from intercurrent disease died from myocardial infarction, compared to no intercurrent deaths in the treated group [93]. Two other observational studies support the contention that oestrogen is not harmful to postmenopausal women [94,95].

The American College of Obstetricians and Gynecologists [96] stated that, "in women with a history of endometrial cancer, oestrogens could be used for the same indications as for any other woman except that the selection of appropriate candidates should be based on prognostic indicators and the risk the patient is willing to assume."

Whether a progestin should be used in combination with oestrogen in these patients is questionable. Most authors conclude that the addition of progestin to oestrogen seems reasonable and prudent in order to abrogate any stimulatory effect on a hypothetical occult metastatic focus. The most effective dose of progestin to add to the regimen is unknown: in order to achieve the best compliance a possible recommendation is that the patient receive conjugated oestrogen 0.625 mg and medroxyprogesterone acetate 2.5 mg daily according to a continuous combined schedule.

Although no prospective randomised trials on ERT or HRT after primary therapy for endometrial cancer have been reported to date, there are several factors suggesting that hormones may, and probably should, be given in a large majority of women with a history of endometrial cancer [97]. The great majority of endometrial cancers are stage I and II and are therefore curable by appropriate surgery. If no pelvic nodes are involved at surgery, the long-term survival is more than 80%.

If a woman with stage I-II, node-negative endometrial cancer becomes post-menopausal as a result of surgery, there is a great risk that she will suffer severe morbidity as a result of oestrogen deficiency; for example, she will have a three times higher risk of osteoporotic fractures and cardiovascular disease than a healthy woman. Women with advanced stage endometrial cancer have a poor prognosis in spite of salvage surgery, radiotherapy and/or chemotherapy. One way to improve the length and quality of life is to administer a progestogen and add an oestrogen if the menopausal symptoms persist.

Cervical cancer

Carcinoma of the cervix, even in preinvasive forms, is not directly influenced by oestrogens or other hormone therapy. In fact, squamous cell carcinoma of the cervix does not respond to oestrogens and ERT has therefore no adverse effect on the outcome of the disease [98]. This observation has led to the recommendation to preserve the ovaries in young patients at the time of initial treatment. In postmenopausal patients ERT may be beneficial in alleviating dyspareunia due to vaginal irradiation therapy and in decreasing the frequency and severity of intestinal and bladder complications, resulting in a better quality of life [99].

Adenocarcinoma of the endocervix may be influenced by hormones: there is, however, no clear evidence that the use of oestrogens has induced any adverse growth when administered to patients with previous adenocarcinoma of the cervix. Until prospective studies will clarify this issue, it could be recommended to treat these women as if they had adenocarcinoma of the endometrium [98].

Carcinoma of the vagina

This neoplasm is a rare disease, accounting for 1-2% of all gynaecological cancers. The presence of oestrogen and progesterone receptors as well as the response of the vaginal epithelium to sex hormones during the menstrual cycle are well documented, but there are no clinical or experimental data to suggest that these hormones are associated with the development of primary or recurrent vaginal cancer. HRT appears to be safe and may even be beneficial for tumour control [98].

Carcinoma of the vulva

Carcinoma of the vulva represents about 5% of all gynaecological cancers, with most cases occurring in postmenopausal patients. This neoplasm does not respond to oestrogen or progesterone, probably because squamous cells are usually not directly stimulated by female sex hormones; as a consequence, HRT has no adverse effect on the outcome of this disease [98].

Ovarian cancer

Epithelial ovarian cancer is not considered a hormone-related disease; a history of epithelial ovarian cancer is therefore no contraindication to HRT. Many studies have been conducted on the risk of ovarian cancer among postmenopausal women during or after HRT; most of them showed no significant association, the relative risk being 1.1 (95% confidence interval 0.6-2) [100]. Two case-control [101,102] and one prospective study [103] showed a significant risk increase in women treated with long-term HRT, but a meta-analysis of over 2000 cases and 8000 controls in the USA did not: the pooled relative risk of cancer for ever HRT users was 0.9 in hospital-based studies and 1.1 in population-based ones, without any effect of the duration of treatment [104].

Data concerning the safety of HRT following the diagnosis of ovarian cancer are scarce. Although many ovarian cancers express oestrogen and progesterone receptors, this observation does not necessarily suggest that these receptors are functional except, perhaps, in well-differentiated endometrioid carcinomas [105,106]. It could be expected that endometrioid epithelial ovarian tumours might respond to hormones; nevertheless, in spite of the presence of hormone receptors, there is no evidence that the growth of these tumours is influenced by HRT.

The only study on the role of HRT following ovarian cancer treatment is a retrospective one by Eeles et al. [107]: this study showed no significant difference in overall and disease-free survival between 78 women who underwent HRT following ovarian cancer therapy and 295 women who were not treated, after accounting for the effects of other prognostic factors (stage of disease, grade of differentiation, histotype, and time to relapse). Although the numbers were small, HRT improved the survival of patients with endometrioid and clear cell cancer. This paper suggests that HRT does not have any adverse effects in patients treated for carcinoma of the ovary.

A recent reanalysis of the European studies found that HRT may have a weak promoting effect on ovarian carcinogenesis. However, the authors acknowledge that the association may reflect selective administration to high-risk individuals [108].

Prospective, randomised studies are needed to evaluate the safety of HRT in this category of patients; at present there appears to be no contraindication to HRT in women previously treated for epithelial ovarian cancer.

Gestational trophoblastic neoplasia

There are no published data on the role of HRT in women previously treated for this disease. Information may be obtained from indirect observations regarding many of its aspects. No study has ever demonstrated oestrogen or progesterone to be part of the aetiology of gestational trophoblastic neoplasia: the neoplasm is associated with genetic conception anomalies. Most of the patients treated for this disease retain their ovaries and are therefore exposed to normal hormone levels: this has never been associated with a worse survival. Several publications have reported pregnancies following primary treatment without significant reactivation of the disease [109-111]. These indirect observations suggest that HRT is safe in women previously treated for gestational trophoblastic neoplasia.

Sarcomas

There is a dearth of information about the incidence of primary or recurrent sarcomas in patients on HRT. This is hardly surprising, as these diseases are extremely uncommon (less than 1% of all cancers) and it would be very difficult to detect an increased risk during HRT. Epidemiological findings have shown that women have a better survival than men and that sarcomas occurring in premenopause appear to be associated with a remarkably better survival (10-year survival rate 50% versus 30%) than those occurring in postmenopausal or premenarcheal years [112]. Analyses of the steroid receptor content in the different types of sarcomas show that most of them lack oestrogen and progesterone receptor proteins [113]. This and other observations may suggest that the female hormone environment influences the natural history of these tumours.

There are not many data showing that oestrogenic stimulation alters the outcome of patients treated for genital tract sarcomas: an anedoctal experience from Yale-New Haven Medical Center suggests that use of HRT in low-grade endometrial stromal sarcomas (the so-called endolymphatic stromal myosis) may be associated with recurrence of disease [114]. Fox reported a case of an early recurrence in a woman who had been treated by hysterectomy and bilateral salpingo-oophorectomy for an endometrial stromal sarcoma and subsequently underwent HRT [115]. This clinical experience may be confirmed by the evidence that this very rare type of neoplasia often contains high levels of oestrogen and progestin receptors and is sensitive to HRT, although the receptor status of a sarcoma does not appear to be of prognostic significance [116].

Thus, with the exception of this tumour, HRT is very unlikely to be of prognostic significance in patients treated for soft tissue sarcomas.

Colorectal cancer

Colorectal cancer is the second most common cancer in women in developed countries and the third leading cause of cancer death in women. More than 30 studies have been reported on the use of HRT in patients treated for colorectal cancer. Most of the studies and two recent meta-analyses found a protective effect of HRT against the development of colorectal cancer, with an overall protection in long-term HRT users of 30-40% [117-122]. The protection might be due to the effect of female hormones on bile acid secretion and synthesis or to a direct effect on the colonic mucosa.

Although the majority of studies, especially the more rigorously designed recent studies, support the conclusion that postmenopausal ERT has a protective effect against colorectal cancer, methodological limitations currently preclude the practical application of the study results. Confirmation by prospective studies that HRT protects against colorectal carcinogenesis would have a major public health impact due to the frequency and high mortality of this disease.

Liver cancer

There are some data that support a potentially favourable impact of HRT on liver cancer. A Swedish record-linked study reports a mortality ratio of 0.4 among patients who underwent HRT [123]. In an Italian case-control study the risk of liver cancer was confirmed to be below 1.0 [124] and no association between hepatocellular carcinoma and use of oestrogens was observed in another case-control study from Los Angeles County [125].

Gastric cancer

There are no epidemiological findings to suggest that reproductive factors are of any importance in the pathogenesis of gastric cancer, nor is there convincing evidence that female sex hormone receptors, which are present in most gastric carcinomas, play a role in gastric carcinogenesis [126].

Conclusions

The benefits of HRT are well known, including the relief of postmenopausal symptoms, the prevention of osteoporosis and coronary heart disease, and the long-term beneficial effects on the central nervous system. Many women entering menopause have significant vasomotor and urogenital symptoms, and restriction of the benefits of oestrogen does not appear to be appropriate. Moreover, many cancer patients risk more potential problems with osteoporosis and cardiovascular disease than with recurrence of their cancer. Given the recent data it may be worthwhile to re-evaluate the usual recommendations, especially when replacement therapy consists of both oestrogen and progestin. The decision to prescribe HRT to postmenopausal women should be taken only after a thorough evaluation of the clinical status of the patient and the risks and benefits of such therapy.

Hormonal therapy following cancer is not contraindicated for the majority of women. Vulvar cancer, vaginal cancer, squamous cell carcinoma of the cervix, gestational trophoblastic neoplasia, genital tract sarcomas (except for the endometrial stromal histotype), gastric cancer and melanoma are not influenced by hormones. Many observations suggest that HRT is effective in the prevention of colorectal cancer. There are no data to support the assumption that combined oestrogen-progestogen treatment is contraindicated in patients who have had endometrial cancer or adenocarcinoma of the uterine cervix. As far as ovarian cancer is concerned, there is no evidence from the literature that HRT is detrimental following treatment for this neoplasm. This is further supported by the observation that patients with stage I epithelial ovarian cancers who have retained ovarian function have a similar prognosis to those who were surgically castrated as part of their treatment.

It has been common practice to prohibit HRT in patients treated for breast cancer. The reappraisal of this practice is mandatory because the beneficial role of HRT in preventing coronary artery disease and osteoporosis and in improving quality of life is well established. A small number of studies have found a slightly increased risk of developing breast cancer in specific subgroups of patients using ERT. However, in all studies the risk incidence was minimal or of borderline significance. Since 1980 more than 50 case-control studies, cohort studies and formal meta-analyses have been unable to provide substantial evidence regarding this very important issue; the effects of biases can only be eliminated by large, randomised studies such as the ongoing Women's Health Initiative in the US (to be completed in 2008) and the WISDOM trial (Women's International Study of Long-Duration Oestrogen use after Menopause) in the UK (to be completed in 2011). Patients must be aware of the possibility of a recurrence coinciding with any new hormone exposure, because freedom from recurrent breast cancer can never be guaranteed.

While it is generally accepted that hormone replacement taken for five years or less does not increase the risk of breast cancer, when the long-term use (more than 10-15 years) is considered some authors have found a small increase in the risk, possibly limited to women who are currently receiving HRT or who have recently stopped such therapy. This would translate into an increase in the absolute risk of developing breast cancer of 3% to 4%. It has been estimated that the cumulative excess breast cancer incidence in 1000 women who used HRT for 10 years, beginning at age 50, is 6 [127].

There is no evidence suggesting that hormone therapy is contraindicated in women with a history of benign breast disease. The epidemiological data indicate that a positive family history of breast cancer should not be a contraindication to the use of HRT. No evidence exists on differing risks of breast cancer with different types of oestrogens, and no clear dose relationship has been found. There is no clear evidence of a protective effect of the addition of a progestogen.

Death from any cause in current HRT users is reduced by 30% compared with non-users. This refers not only to the protective effects against cardiovascular and bone disease, but also to the less virulent cancers arising in women who have taken HRT [80,81,128-130]. It is also remarkable that the mortality of all malignancies is reduced and the mortality of colon cancer is reduced by 50% in HRT users compared with non-users.

An analysis of the risks and benefits of HRT is therefore recommended. Whilst one in 8-12 women may contract breast cancer in the Western world, one in three women over 65 years of age will have cardiovascular disease and 30-50% of postmenopausal women will have osteoporosis [131].

Harlap [132] noted that ERT results in an excess mortality from breast and endometrial cancer of 38 in 100,000 and 26 in 100,000, respectively. The combined decrease in mortality from stroke, heart disease and hip fractures in oestrogen users was calculated to be 366 out of 100,000, with an overall benefit among women in the 65 to 74 year age group of between 302 and 328 out of 100,000 in prevention of death [133]. The combination of oestrogen plus progesterone was estimated to reduce this benefit to 211 in 100,000 women by its effect on cardio-vascular mortality [132]. A recent study by Ross et al. concludes that the benefits of HRT appear to outweigh the risks: for each incident case of breast cancer due to long-term use of HRT more than six deaths from heart disease are prevented [134]. On the basis of these data many women will realise that the benefits outweigh the risks, even following treatment for an oestrogen-related neoplasm.

References

1   Cummings SR, Kelsey JL, Nevitt NC, O'Dowd KJ. Epidemiology of osteoporosis and osteoporotic fractures. Epidemiol Rev 1986; 7: 178-208

2   Stempfer MJ, Colditz GA. Estrogen replacement therapy and coronary heart disease: quantitative assessment of the epidemiologic evidence. Prev Med 1991; 273: 47-63

3   Schairer C, Adami HO, Hoover R, Persson I. Cause-specific mortality in women receiving hormone replacement therapy. Epidemiology 1997; 8: 59-65

4   Henderson VW, Paganini-Hill A, Emanuel CK, et al. Estrogen replacement therapy in older women. Arch Neurol 1994; 51: 896-900

5   Okhura T, Isse K, Akazawa K, et al. Long-term estrogen replacement therapy in female patients with dementia of the Alzheimer type: 7 case reports. Dementia 1995; 6: 99-107

6   Samsoie G. Urogenital aging: a hidden problem. Am J Obstet Gynecol 1998; 178: 245-9

7   Brincat M, Galea R, Muscat Baron Y, Cardozo L. Effect of the menopause on skin and urogenital tissue. Eur Menopause J 1996; 3: 237-41

8   World Health Organization. Assessment of fracture risk and its application to screening for postmenopausal osteoporosis. WHO Technical Report Series 1994; 843

9   Slemenda C, Hui SL, Longcope C, Johnston CC. Sex steroids and bone mass: a study of changes about the time of menopause. J Clin Invest 1987; 80: 1261-9

10   National Osteoporosis Foundation. Osteoporosis: Physician's guide to prevention and treatment of osteoporosis. Belle Mead, NJ: Excerpta Medica, 1998

11   Riggs BL, Melton LJ. The prevention and treatment of osteoporosis. N Engl J Med 1992; 327: 620-7

12   Lindsay R. Prevention and treatment of osteoporosis. Lancet 1993; i: 801-5

13   Grady D, Rubin SM, Petitti DB, et al. Hormone therapy to prevent disease and prolong life in postmenopausal women. Ann Intern Med 1992; 117: 1016-37

14   Hutchinson TA, Polanski SM, Feinstein AR. Postmenopausal oestrogens protect against fractures of hip and distal radius. Lancet 1979; ii: 705-9

15   Weiss SR, Ellman H, Dolker M, for the Transdermal Estradiol Investigator Group. A randomized controlled trial of four doses of transdermal estradiol for preventing postmenopausal bone loss. Obstet Gynecol 1999; 94: 330-6

16   Paganini-Hill A, Ross RK, Gerkins VR, et al. Menopausal estrogen therapy and hip fractures. Ann Intern Med 1981; 95: 28-31

17   Kiel DP, Felson DT, Anderson JJ, et al. Hip fracture and the use of estrogens in post-menopausal women: the Framingham study. N Engl J Med 1987; 317: 1169-74

18   Ettinger B, Grady D. The waning effect of postmenopausal estrogen therapy on osteoporosis. N Engl J Med 1993; 329: 1192-3

19   World Health Organization. World Health Statistics Annual. Geneva: WHO, 1988

20   Eaker ED, Chesbro JH, Sacks FM, et al. Cardiovascular disease in women. Circulation 1993; 88: 1999-2009

21   Grodstein F, Stampter MJ, Manson JE, et al. Postmenopausal estrogen and progestin use and the risk of cardiovascular disease. N Engl J Med 1996; 335: 453-61

22   Rosano GM, Panina G. Cardiovascular pharmacology of hormone replacement therapy. Drugs Aging 1999; 15: 219-34

23   Clemente C, Caruso MG, Berloco P, et al. Antioxidant effect of short-term hormonal treatment in postmenopausal women. Maturitas 1999; 31: 137-42

24   Stevenson JC, Crook D, Godsland IF. Effect of age and menopause on lipid metabolism in healthy women. Atherosclerosis 1993; 98: 83-90

25   Assman G, Cullen P, Schulte H. HRT, plasma risk factors and cardiovascular disease. Eur Menopause 1996; 3: 203-8

26   Hulley S, Grady D, Bush T, et al. Randomized trial of estrogen plus progestin for secondary prevention of coronary heart disease in postmenopausal women. JAMA 1998; 280: 605-13

27   Barrett-Connor E, Stuenkel C. Hormones and heart disease in women: Heart and Estrogen/progestin Replacement Study in perspective. J Clin Endocrinol Metab 1999; 84: 1848-53

28   Mijatovic V, van der Mooren MJ, Stehouwer CD, et al. Postmenopausal hormone replacement, risk estimators for coronary heart disease and cardiovascular protection. Gynecol Endocrinol 1999; 13: 130-44

29   Fung MM, Barrett-Connor E, Bettencourt RR. Hormone replacement therapy and stroke risk in postmenopausal women. J Women's Health 1999; 8: 359-64

30   Ross RK, Pike MC, Henderson BE, et al. Stroke prevention and oestrogen replacement therapy. Lancet 1989; 1: 505

31   Finucane FF, Madans JH, Bush TL. Decreased risk of stroke among postmenopausal hormone users. Results from a national cohort. Arch Intern Med 1993; 153: 73-9

32   McEwen BS, Alves BS. Estrogen actions in the central nervous system. Endocrin Rev 1999; 20: 279-307

33   Chung SK, Pfaff DK, Cohen RS. Estrogen-induced alterations in synaptic morphology in the midbrain central grey. Exp Brain Res 1988; 69: 522-30

34   Brinton RD, Tran J, Proffitt P, et al. 17beta estradiol enhances the outgrowth and survival of neocortical neurons in culture. Neurochem Res 1997; 22: 1339-51

35   Goodman Y, Bruce AJ, Cheng B, et al. Estrogens attenuate and corticosterone exacerbates excitotoxicity, oxidative injury, and amyloid beta-peptide toxicity in hippocampal neurons. J Neurochem 1996; 66: 1836-44

36   Panay N, Studd JW. The psychotherapeutic effects of estrogens. Gynecol Endocrinol 1998; 12: 353-65

37   Poirier J. Apolipoprotein E in animal models of CNS injury and in Alzheimer's disease. Trends Neurosci 1994; 17: 525-80

38   Boyles JK, Zoellner CD, Anderson JL, et al. A role for apolipoprotein E, apolipoprotein A-I, and low density lipoprotein receptors in cholesterol transport during regeneration and remyelination of the rat sciatic nerve. J Clin Invest 1989; 83: 1015-31

39   Birge SJ. Practical strategies for the diagnosis and treatment of Alzheimer's disease. Clinical Geriatrics 1999; 7: 56-74

40   Tang MX, Jacobs D, Stern Y, et al. Effect of oestrogen during menopause on risk and age at onset of Alzheimer's disease. Lancet 1996; 348: 429-32

41   Slooter AJC, Bronzova J, Witteman JCM, et al. Oestrogen use and early onset Alzheimer's disease: a population based study. J Neurol Neurosurg Psychiatry 1999; 67: 779-81

42   van Duijn CM. Hormone replacement therapy and Alzheimer's disease. Maturitas 1999; 31: 201-5

43   Waring SC, Rocca WA, Petersen RC, et al. Postmenopausal estrogen replacement therapy and risk of AD: a population-based study. Neurology 1999; 52: 965-70

44   Paganini-Hill A, Henderson VW. Estrogen replacement therapy and risk of Alzheimer's disease. Arch Intern Med 1996; 156: 2213-7

45   Brenner D, Kukull VA, Stergachis A, et al. Postmenopausal estrogen replacement therapy and the risk of Alzheimer's disease: a population-based case-control study. Am J Epidemiol 1994; 140: 262-7

46   Kawas C, Resnick S, Morrison A, et al. A prospective study of estrogen replacement therapy and the risk of developing Alzheimer's disease: the Baltimore Longitudinal Study of Aging. Neurology 1997; 48: 1517-21

47   Fillit H, Weinreb H, Cholst I, et al. Observations in a preliminary open trial of estradiol therapy for senile dementia – Alzheimer's type. Psychoneuroendocrinology 1986; 11: 337-45

48   Honjo H, Ogino Y, Naitoh K, et al. In vivo effects by estrone sulfate on the central nervous system: senile dementia (Alzheimer's type). J Steroid Biochem 1989; 34: 521-5

49   Okhura T, Isse K, Akazawa K, et al. Evaluation of estrogen treatment in female patients with dementia of the Alzheimer type. Endocrinol J 1994; 41: 361-71

50   Ashtana S, Craft S, Baker LD, et al. Cognitive and neuroendocrine response to transdermal estrogen in postmenopausal women with Alzheimer's disease: result of a placebo-controlled, double-blind pilot study. Psychoneuroendocrinology 1999; 24: 657-77

51   Steffens DC, Notelovitz M, Plassman BL, et al. Enhanced cognitive performance with estrogen use in non-demented community-dwelling older women. J Am Geriatr Soc 1999; 47: 1171-5

52   Jacobs D, Tang MX, Stern Y, et al. Cognitive function in non-demented older women who took estrogen after menopause. Neurol 1998; 50: 368-73

53   Barrett-Connor E, Kritz-Silverstein D. Estrogen replacement therapy and cognitive function in older women. JAMA 1993; 269: 2637-41

54   Matthews K, Cauley J, Yaffe K, et al. Estrogen replacement therapy and cognitive decline in older community women. J Am Geriatr Soc 1999; 47: 518-23

55   Kampen DL, Sherwin BB. Estrogen use and verbal memory in healthy postmenopausal women. Obstet Gynecol 1994; 83: 979-83

56   Kimura D. Estrogen replacement therapy may protect against intellectual decline in postmenopausal women. Horm Behav 1995: 29: 312-21

57   Blanchet PJ, Fang J, Hylan K, Arnold LA, Mouradian MM, Chase TN. Short-term effects of high-dose 17beta-estradiol in postmenopausal PD patients: a cross-over study. Neurology 1999; 53: 91-5

58   Saunders-Pullman R, Gordon-Elliott J, Parides M, et al. The effect of estrogen replacement on early Parkinson's disease. Neurology 1999; 52: 1417-21

59   Evans JR, Schwartz SD, McHugh JD, et al. Systemic factors for idiopathic macular holes: a case-control study. Eye 1998; 12: 256-9

60   Metka M, Enzelsberger H, Knogler W, et al. Ophthalmic complaints as a climacteric symptom. Maturitas 1991; 14: 3-9

61   Vingerling JR, Dielemans I, Witteman CM, et al. Macular degeneration and early menopause: a case-control study. BMJ 1995; 310: 1570-1

62   Col NF, Eckman MH, Karas RH, et al. Patient-specific decisions about hormone replacement therapy in postmenopausal women. JAMA 1997; 277: 1140-7

63   Ribeiro G, Jones DA, Jones M. Carcinoma of the breast associated with pregnancy. Br J Surg 1986; 73: 607-9

64   King RM, Welch JS, Martin JK Jr. Carcinoma of the breast associated with pregnancy. Surg Gynecol Obstet 1985; 160: 228-32

65   Mignot L, Morvan F, Berdah J, et al. Grossesses après cancer du sein traité. Resultats d'une étude cas-témoins. Presse Med 1986; 15: 1961-4

66   Cooper DR, Butterfield J. Pregnancy subsequent to mastectomy for cancer of the breast. Ann Surg 1970; 171: 429-33

67   Clark RM, Reid J. Carcinoma of the breast in pregnancy and lactation. Int J Radiat Oncol Biol Phys 1978; 4: 693-8

68   Rosner D, Lane W. Oral contraceptive use has no adverse effect on the prognosis of breast cancer. Cancer 1986; 57: 591-6

69   Ravdin RG, Lewison EF, Slack NH, et al. Results of a clinical trial concerning the worth of prophylactic oophorectomy for breast carcinoma. Surg Gynecol Obstet 1970; 131: 1055-64

70   Nachtigall MJ, Smilen SW, Nachtigall RD, Nachtigall RH, Nachtigall LI. Incidence of breast cancer in a 22-year study of women receiving estrogen-progestin replacement therapy. Obstet Gynecol 1992; 80: 827-30

71   Armstrong BK. Oestrogen therapy after the menopause: boon or bane? Med J Aust 1988; 148: 213-4

72   Dupont VD, Page DL. Menopausal estrogen replacement therapy and breast cancer. Arch Intern Med 1991; 151: 67-72

73   Steinberg KK, Thacker SB, Smith SJ, et al. A meta-analysis of the effect of estrogen replacement therapy on the risk of breast cancer. JAMA 1991; 265: 1985-90

74   Sillero-Arenas M, Delgado-Rodriguez M, Rodigues-Canteras R, Bueno-Cavanillas A, Galvez-Fargas R. Menopausal hormone replacement therapy and breast cancer: a meta-analysis. Obstet Gynecol 1992; 79: 286-94

75   Colditz GA, Egan KM, Stampfer MJ. Hormone replacement therapy and risk of breast cancer: results from epidemiologic studies. Am J Obstet Gynecol 1993; 168: 1473-80

76   Grady D, Rubin SM, Petitti DB, et al. Hormone therapy to prevent disease and prolong life in postmenopausal women. Ann Intern Med 1992; 117: 1016-37

77   Colditz GA, Hankinson SE, Hunter DJ, et al. The use of estrogens and progestins and risk of breast cancer in postmenopausal women. N Engl J Med 1995; 335: 1589-93

78   Grodstein F, Stempfer MJ, Colditz GA, et al. Postmenopausal hormone therapy and mortality. N Engl J Med 1997; 336: 1769-75

79   Collaborative Group on Hormonal Factors in Breast Cancer. Breast cancer and hormone replacement therapy. Lancet 1997; 350: 1047-59

80   Magnusson C, Baron JA, Correia N, et al. Breast cancer risk following long-term oestrogen and oestrogen-progestin replacement therapy. Int J Cancer 1999; 81: 339-44

81   Gapstur SM, Morrow M, Sellars TA. Hormone replacement therapy and the risk of breast cancer with a favorable histology: results of the Iowa Women's Health Study. JAMA 1999; 281: 2091-7

82   Lando JF, Heck KE, Brett KM. Hormone replacement therapy and breast cancer risk in a nationally representative cohort. Am J Prev Med 1999; 17: 176-80

83   Lobo RA. Hormone replacement therapy/oestrogen replacement after treatment for breast cancer? Lancet 1993; 341: 1313-4

84   DiSaia PJ, Odicino F, Grosen EA, Cowan B, Pecorelli S, Wile AG. Hormone replacement therapy in breast cancer [letter]. Lancet 1993; 342: 232

85   Di Saia PJ, Grosen EA, Kurosaki T, Gildea M, Cowan B, Anton-Culver H. Hormone replacement therapy in breast cancer survivors: a cohort study. Am J Obstet Gynecol 1996; 174: 494-8

86   Powles C. Hormone replacement therapy after breast cancer [letter]. Lancet 1993; 342: 60-1

87   Stoll BA, Parbhoo S. Treatment of menopausal symptoms in breast cancer patients. Lancet 1988; i: 1278-9

88 Wile AG, Opfell RW, Margileth DA. Hormone replacement in previously treated breast cancer patients. Am J Surg 1993; 165: 372-5

89 Eden JA, Bush T, Nand S, Wren BG. A case-control study of combined continuous estrogen-progestin replacement therapy among women with a personal history of breast cancer. Menopause 1995; 2: 67-72

90 Vassilopoulou-Sellin R, Theriault R, Klein MJ. Estrogen replacement therapy in women with prior diagnosis and treatment for breast cancer. Gynecol Oncol 1997; 65: 89-93

91 Vassilopoulou-Sellin R, Asmar L, Hortobagyi GN, et al. Estrogen replacement therapy after localized breast cancer: clinical outcome of 319 women followed prospectively. J Clin Oncol 1999; 17: 1482-7

92 Creasman WT, Henderson D, Hinshaw W, Clarke-Pearson BL. Estrogen replacement therapy in the patient treated for endometrial cancer. Obstet Gynecol 1986; 647: 326-30

93 Lee RB, Burke TW, Park RC. Estrogen replacement therapy following treatment for stage I endometrial cancer. Gynaecol Oncol 1990; 36: 189-91

94 Baker DD. Estrogen replacement therapy in patients with previous endometrial carcinoma. Comp Ther 1990; 16: 28-35

95 Bryant GW. Administration of estrogen to patients with a previous diagnosis of endometrial adenocarcinoma. South Med J 1990; 83: 725-6

96 ACOG Committee Opinion, Number 80, February 1990

97 Burger CW, van Leeuwen FE, Scheele F, et al. Hormone replacement therapy in women treated for gynecologic malignancy. Maturitas 1999; 32: 69-76

98 Wren BG. Hormonal therapy following female genital tract cancer. Int J Gynecol Cancer 1994; 4: 217-24

99 Ploch E. Hormonal replacement therapy in patients after cervical cancer treatment. Gynecol Oncol 1987; 26: 169-77

100 Pejovic-Lenfant MH. Risque carcinologique des traitements hormonaux substitutifs de la ménopause. J Gynec Obstet Biol Reprod 1989; 18: 153-6

101 Polychronopoulou A, Tzonou A, Hsieh CC, et al. Reproductive variables, tobacco, ethanol, coffee and somatometry as risk factors for ovarian cancer. Int J Cancer 1993; 55: 402-7

102 Parazzini F, La Vecchia C, Negri E, Villa A. Estrogen replacement therapy and ovarian cancer risk. Int J Cancer 1994; 57: 135-6

103 Rodriguez C, Calle EE, Coates RJ, Miracle-McMahill HL, Thun MJ, Heath CW Jr. Estrogen replacement therapy and fatal ovarian cancer. Am J Epidemiol 1995; 141: 828-35

104 Whittemore AS, Harris R, Itnyre J. Characteristics relating to ovarian cancer risk: collaborative analysis of 12 US case-control studies. II. Invasive epithelial ovarian cancers in white women. Collaborative Ovarian Cancer Group. Am J Epidemiol 1992; 136: 1184-203

105 Schwartz PE, Naftolin F. Hormone therapy. In: Berek JS, Hacker NF, eds. Practical gynecologic oncology. Baltimore: Williams & Wilkins 1994; 613-36

106 Rendina GM, Donadio C, Giovannini M. Steroid receptors and progestinic therapy in ovarian endometrioid carcinoma. Eur J Gynaecol Oncol 1982; 3: 241-6

107 Eeles RA, Tan S, Wiltshaw E, et al. Hormone replacement therapy and survival after surgery for ovarian cancer. Br Med J 1991; 302: 259-62

108 Negri E, Tzounou A, Beral V, et al. Hormonal therapy for menopause and ovarian cancer in a collaborative reanalysis of European studies. Int J Cancer 1999; 80: 848-51

109 Ngan HY, Wong LC, Ma HK. Reproductive performance of patients with gestational trophoblastic disease in Hong Kong. Acta Obstet Gynecol Scand 1988; 67: 11-4

110 Ayhan A, Ergeneli MH, Yuce K, Yappar EG, Kisnisci AH. Pregnancy after chemotherapy for gestational trophoblastic disease. J Reprod Med 1990; 35: 522-4

111 DeMola L Jr, Goldfarb JM. Reproductive performance of patients after gestational trophoblastic disease. Sem Oncol 1995; 22: 193-7

112 Cantin J, McNeer GP. The effect of pregnancy on the clinical course of sarcoma of the soft somatic tissues. Surg Gynecol Obstet 1967; 125: 28-32

113 Chaudhuri PK, Walker MJ, Beattie CW, Das Gupta TK. Distribution of steroid hormone receptors in human soft tissue sarcomas. Surgery 1981; 90: 149-52

114 Horowitz K, Rutherford T, Schwartz PE. Hormone replacement therapy in women with sarcomas. CME J Gynec Oncol 1996; 1: 23-9

115 Fox H. Hormone replacement therapy and sarcoma. CME J Gynec Oncol 1996; 1: 30-1

116 Wade K, Quinn MA, Hammond I, Williams K, Cauchi M. Uterine sarcoma: steroid receptors and response to hormonal therapy. Gynecol Oncol 1990; 39: 364-7

117 Clinical Synthesis Panel on HRT. Hormone replacement therapy. Lancet 1999; 354: 152-5

118 Franceschi S, La Vecchia C. Colorectal cancer and hormone replacement therapy: an unexpected finding. Eur J Cancer Prev 1998; 7: 427-38

119 Calle EE, Miracle-McMahill HL, Thun MJ, Heath CW Jr. Estrogen replacement therapy and risk of fatal colon cancer in a prospective cohort of postmenopausal women. J Natl Cancer Inst 1995; 87: 517-23

120 Fernandez E, La Vacchia C, D'Avanzo B, et al. Oral contraceptives, hormone replacement therapy and the risk of colorectal cancer. Br J Cancer 1996; 73: 1431-5

121 Nanda K, Bastian LA, Hasselbald V, Simel DL. Hormone replacement therapy and the risk of colorectal cancer: a meta-analysis. Obstet Gynecol 1999; 93: 880-8

122 Grodstein F, Newcomb PA, Stampfer MJ. Postmenopausal hormone therapy and risk of colorectal cancer: a review and meta-analysis. Am J Med 1999; 106: 574-82

123 Adami H-O, Persson I, Hoover R, Schairer C, Bergkvist L. Risk of cancer in women receiving hormone replacement therapy. Int J Cancer 1989; 44: 833-9

124 Tavani A, Negri E, Parazzini F, et al. Female hormone utilization and risk of hepatocellular carcinoma. Br J Cancer 1993; 67: 635-7

125 Yu MC, Tong MJ, Govindarajan S, Henderson BE. Nonviral risk factors for hepatocellular carcinoma in a low-risk population, the non-Asians of Los Angeles County, California. J Natl Cancer Inst 1991; 83: 1820-6

126 Hunt K, Vessey M, McPherson K. Mortality in a cohort of long-term users of hormone replacement therapy: an updated analysis. Br J Obstet Gynaecol 1990; 97: 1080-6

127 Beral V, Banks E, Reeves G, Appleby P. Use of HRT and the subsequent risk of cancer. J Epidemiol Biostat 1999; 4: 191-210

128 Strickland DM, Gambrell RD, Butzin CA, Strickland K. The relationship between breast cancer survival and prior postmenopausal estrogen use. Obstet Gynecol 1992; 80: 400-4

129 Squitieri R, Tartter PI, Ahmed S, Brower ST, Theise ND. Carcinoma of the breast in postmenopausal hormone users and non-user controls. J Am Coll Surg 1994; 178: 167-70

130 Bonnier P, Romain S, Giacaione PL, Laffargue F, Martin PM, Piana L. Clinical and biological prognostic factors in breast cancer diagnosed during postmenopausal hormone replacement therapy. Obstet Gynecol 1995; 85: 11-7

131 Schneider HP. HRT and cancer risk: separating facts from fiction. Maturitas 1999; 33 (suppl 1): 65-72

132 Harlap S. The benefits and risks of hormone replacement therapy: an epidemiologic overview. Am J Obstet Gynecol 1992; 166: 1986-92

133 Ross RK, Pike MC, Henderson BE, Mack TM, Lobo RA. Stroke prevention and oestrogen replacement therapy [letter]. Lancet 1989; i: 505

134 Ross RK, Paganini-Hill A, Wan PC, Pike MC. Effect of hormone replacement therapy on breast cancer risk: estrogen versus estrogen plus progestin. J Natl Cancer Inst 2000; 92: 328-32

ESO Scientific Updates, Vol. 5
Fatigue and Cancer
M. Marty and S. Pecorelli, editors

Radiotherapy-Induced Fatigue

Barbara A. Jereczek-Fossa[1,2], Hugo Raul Marsiglia[1] and Roberto Orecchia[1,3]

1   Department of Radiotherapy, European Institute of Oncology, Milan, Italy
2   Department of Oncology and Radiotherapy, Medical University of Gdansk, Poland
3   University of Milan, Italy

Introduction

Fatigue is one of the most common symptoms reported by cancer patients. Despite its high prevalence and serious adverse effects on quality of life (QOL), this symptom is underestimated by medical and nursing staff [1]. Knowledge of the reasons for fatigue, its correlates, epidemiology and therapeutic management is extremely limited. The published reports are mainly descriptive and in many of them numerous methodological biases are present.

Cancer treatments such as surgery, chemotherapy, radiation therapy or biological response modifiers often induce fatigue and tiredness. According to Simon and Zittoun [2] fatigue is becoming a major complaint in a majority of patients, probably due to improved control of other important cancer symptoms such as pain and nausea. Thus it can have major implications for decisions regarding therapy such as the interruption of treatment or dose reduction. In many analyses patients felt that fatigue adversely affected QOL more than pain, sexual dysfunction or other cancer or therapy-related symptoms [1,3-5].

Radiotherapy induces fatigue in up to 80% of patients and in some cases it can persist long after treatment has finished [3,6-8]. Since about 50% of cancer patients receive either curative or palliative radiation therapy during the course of their disease, about 40% of all oncological patients will suffer from radiotherapy-induced fatigue. Because of its high prevalence, it is very important that all medical and nursing staff dealing with cancer patients fully understand this symptom.

Address for correspondence: B.A. Jereczek-Fossa, Department of Radiotherapy, European Institute of Oncology, Via Ripamonti 435, 20141 Milan, Italy. Tel.: +39-02-57489607, fax: +39-02-57489036, e-mail: barbara.fossa@ieo.it

Assessment of fatigue

Fatigue is a multidimensional concept with distinct subjective dimensions, e.g. sensory, emotional and cognitive [2,9]. Assessment of fatigue by single items in general symptom checklists has contributed to underestimation of fatigue in many studies [2]. Recently, modern tools have been designed to measure fatigue. One of them is the multidimensional fatigue inventory (MFI-20), which was tested on a Dutch and Scottish sample of cancer patients receiving radiotherapy [10]. This 20-item self-report measure covers numerous dimensions including general fatigue, physical fatigue, reduced activity, reduced motivation and mental fatigue (five subscales). Other new measures are the revised Piper Fatigue Scale, the Schwartz Cancer Fatigue Scale, the Fatigue Assessment Questionnaire, the Cancer Linear Analogue Scale and FACT-An [2]. Use of these specific tools is highly recommended in the investigation of radiation-related fatigue.

Causes and correlates

The physical causes of radiotherapy-induced fatigue reported in the literature include anaemia, change in weight, serum interleukins, reverse triiodo-thyronine, decline in neuromuscular efficiency, and pulse change with orthostatic stress, but only change in weight was found to be significantly correlated with fatigue [7,11,12]. Similarly, the association between fatigue and numerous psychological factors has been investigated [3,7,13]. Fatigue was found to correlate with symptom distress, mood disturbance and alterations in usual functional activities [14].

The experience of fatigue seems to depend on treatment-related factors, and gradual increase in fatigue during the course of therapy and reduction in fatigue over weekends when therapy is not applied have been reported [7]. Increase in fatigue with increase of radiotherapy fields and dose has been observed [15-18], although this was not confirmed by other groups [3]. Some authors noticed a reduction of fatigue in the second week of therapy, followed by an increase in the third week and a plateau thereafter, suggesting adaptation of the organism to continuing stress [11]. The degree of fatigue, functional disability and pain before radiotherapy were found to be the best predictors of fatigue at nine-month follow-up [3].

Usually fatigue declines when radiation therapy has been completed, and in some analyses fatigue in disease-free cancer patients does not differ from fatigue in the general population [3]. By contrast, numerous studies reported a high prevalence of long-term fatigue after completion of radiation therapy [19, 20]. In some cases late radiotherapy complications (e.g. chronic dyspnoea or diarrhoea) may contribute to chronic treatment-related fatigue [21]. Age and gender have also been found to correlate with chronic therapy-related fatigue, with males and older patients reporting higher fatigue scores [21, 22]. Addition of chemotherapy to irradiation significantly increases treatment-related fatigue [23]. This additive effect can also be observed in cancer survivors treated with combined modalities [24].

Management of fatigue

Knowledge of the therapeutic options in the management of radiotherapy-induced fatigue is limited. Reduction in fatigue, tension, depression and anger was observed after relaxation therapy performed on outpatients undergoing curative or palliative radiotherapy [25]. Physical exercise was demonstrated in a randomised study to be an effective, convenient and low-cost self-care method that reduced fatigue, anxiety and sleep difficulty, improved physical functioning, and facilitated adaptation during radiation therapy for early breast cancer [26]. Sleep and exercise were together found to be an effective method in the Canadian study [27]. Another effective treatment is group psychotherapy during radiotherapy [28].

Few pharmacological agents have been found to be effective in the management of radiation-related fatigue. Correction of anaemia before or during radiotherapy (blood transfusions, administration of erythropoietin) can be useful when fatigue is accompanied by low haemoglobin levels [29].

Since fatigue is one of the most common long-term side effects of radiotherapy, numerous patients continue to seek information [30]. Support and guidance provided by health care professionals are therefore essential.

Disease-related studies on fatigue

Brain tumours

Fatigue is commonly observed during brain radiotherapy and constitutes the main symptom of the somnolence syndrome following cranial irradiation. A study of the Royal Marsden Hospital, UK, demonstrated a period of drowsiness and fatigue lasting from day 11 to day 21 and from day 31 to day 35 after radiotherapy. Patients treated with accelerated fractionation compared with more conventional fractionation experienced more severe drowsiness and fatigue [31].

Fatigue, headache and memory defects were observed in 30%, 35% and 35%, respectively, of two-year astrocytoma survivors treated with radiation therapy [19]. A higher prevalence of fatigue, depressed mood and cognitive disturbances was observed in low-grade glioma patients treated with radiotherapy when compared to control low-grade haematological malignancy survivors [20]. In one study no changes in fatigue were observed over time in an analysis performed before irradiation (after surgery) and three, six, and twelve months after the completion of radiotherapy for low-grade primary brain tumours [32].

Chronic fatigue along with neurological sequelae and impaired memory were the most common side effects observed in patients undergoing prophylactic cranial irradiation (PCI) for small cell lung cancer (SCLC). The incidence of these complications increases in patients over 60 years old, and in those receiving concomitant chemotherapy or a high total or daily radiation dose [33].

Breast cancer

Fatigue is the most common side effect of localised radiation to the breast [26, 30]. It does not increase linearly with the cumulative radiation dose over time but reflects the adaptation of the organism to stress with an increase in fatigue in the first week, a decrease in the second week, another increase in the third week and a plateau thereafter. Within three weeks from radiotherapy the fatigue diminishes [11].

Some studies suggest that fatigue in breast cancer patients is determined by current physical and psychological distress rather than by the cancer itself and previous therapy. Dyspnoea, insufficient sleep and depression account for about 50% of variance in fatigue [13]. However, these findings have not been confirmed by other authors. Fatigue in breast cancer survivors varies according to the type of previous cancer therapy. Women who received combined therapy have the highest fatigue scores and those who received only radiation the lowest [24].

Urological malignancies

Several studies have been performed to assess fatigue and other side effects of radiotherapy for prostate cancer [4,5,12,30]. As in breast cancer patients, fatigue is the most frequently reported long-term side effect in patients treated with radiotherapy for localised carcinoma of the prostate [30]. In fact, long-term fatigue was as important as lower urinary tract symptoms (LUTS) in influencing QOL after therapy [4]. In the logistic regression performed by Fossa et al. [4] in 379 patients, about 30% of whom received radiotherapy, fatigue and LUTS – but not disturbance in sex life or urinary leakage – were correlated with global QOL. In another analysis published by the same group from Norway [5], general QOL dimensions (fatigue, physical functioning and emotional functioning) were of significantly greater importance for QOL than sexuality and LUTS. In contrast to some other cancers, fatigue in prostate cancer patients may not be the result of depression or sleep disturbances. Physical expression of fatigue may be secondary to a decline in neuromuscular efficiency and enhanced muscle fatigue that is independent of the cardiovascular or psychological status of the patients [12]. Whole-pelvis treatment has been found to induce more significant fatigue and energy loss than small-field or conformal irradiation [18].

Surprisingly, testicular cancer survivors (with about 50% of patients treated with radiotherapy) reported to be less exhausted after a working day and to feel more satisfied with life, stronger and fitter than age-matched controls.

However, a higher incidence of anxiety and depression was observed among these patients [34].

Other pelvic tumours (gynaecological and gastrointestinal tumours)

Irradiation is frequently employed either as curative or adjuvant therapy in many pelvic malignancies. Long-term side effects have been reported both for radiotherapy and other treatment modalities. For example, patients who underwent chemotherapy reported poor role and cognitive functioning and had higher scores of fatigue, nausea, vomiting, constipation and financial problems whereas those who underwent radiation therapy more often complained about flatulence and diarrhoea [35].

Fatigue is frequently reported during pelvic radiotherapy and can significantly contribute to the deterioration of a patient's QOL. It has also been observed in patients undergoing gynaecological intracavitary irradiation (brachytherapy) [36]. Nutritional interventions such as a low-fat and low-lactose diet might prevent acute radiation-induced diarrhoea leading to fatigue [37].

In rectal cancer patients receiving radiotherapy a higher rate of fatigue was observed when radiotherapy was employed in the postoperative rather than preoperative setting [38].

Lymphoma

Several studies on Hodgkin's disease survivors have shown the importance of early and chronic treatment-related fatigue. Interestingly, the majority of long-term survivors felt that early short-term side effects were more, or equally, important as late morbidity with respect to the choice of therapy. Unexpected importance was given by patients to fatigue and weight gain compared to other complications such as infertility and risk of relapse [39].

Analysis of the sociomedical situation of survivors showed a significantly superior global QOL and a lower fatigue score in females than in males. Patients treated with mantle-field irradiation had a higher risk of dyspnoea leading to a higher fatigue score and lower QOL [21].

Head and neck cancer

Numerous cancer-related symptoms are present in patients undergoing radiation treatment for head and neck malignancies. Two parallel studies performed before and six and twelve months after irradiation in laryngeal cancer patients (treated with radiotherapy) [40] and in oral cavity and oropharyngeal cancer patients (treated with surgery with or without radiotherapy) [41] showed significant deterioration of physical functioning, fatigue and worsening of almost all head and neck symptoms except pain and speech, which improved. There was also a high level of depression. Despite deterioration of physical functioning and worsening of symptoms during the first year, improvement of emotional functioning was observed after treatment, a fact which was explained by the authors as a result of adaptation and coping processes.

Lung cancer

Radiotherapy is frequently employed in curative and palliative treatment of lung cancer. In the retrospective analysis of Hickok et al. [8] fatigue was observed in 78% of patients and was not strongly correlated with demographic or disease variables. Although improvement of QOL and many cancer symptoms is frequently observed in patients treated with palliative irradiation, fatigue is usually unaffected by such therapy [42,43].

Bone metastases

About 30% of all cancer patients develop bone metastases during the course of their disease and they are frequently treated with palliative radiotherapy. Pain, fatigue and sleep disturbances are the most common complaints of this patient subgroup. Both external-beam irradiation and radionuclide therapy with strontuim-89 may induce significant fatigue [44,45].

Conclusions

Radiotherapy-induced fatigue is a common, early and chronic side effect of irradiation. It is frequently underestimated by medical and nursing staff and its causes, correlates and prevalence are poorly understood. In numerous analyses the level of fatigue and its time course have been shown to depend on the type of malignancy and treatment modalities. Fatigue may affect global QOL more than pain, sexual dysfunction and other cancer- or treatment-related symptoms. Further methodologically correct studies are warranted to better define the causes, optimal prevention and management of this symptom.

References

1   Vogelzang NJ, Breitbart W, Cella D, et al. Patient, caregiver, and oncologist perceptions of cancer-related fatigue: results of a tripart assessment survey. The Fatigue Coalition. Semin Hematol 1997; 34 (suppl 2): 4-12
2   Simon AM, Zittoun R. Fatigue in cancer patients. Curr Opin Oncol 1999; 11: 244-9
3   Smets EM, Visser MR, Willems-Groot AF, Garssen B, Schuster-Uitterhoeve AL, de Haes JC. Fatigue and radiotherapy: (B) experience in patients 9 months following treatment. Br J Cancer 1998; 78: 907-12
4   Fossa SD, Woehre H, Kurth KH, et al. Influence of urological morbidity on quality of life in patients with prostate cancer. Eur Urol 1997; 31 (suppl 3): 3-8

5   Lilleby W, Fossa SD, Waehre HR, Olsen DR. Long-term morbidity and quality of life in patients with localized prostate cancer undergoing definitive radiotherapy or radical prostatectomy. Int J Radiat Oncol Biol Phys 1999; 43: 735-43

6   Smets EM, Garssen B, Schuster-Uitterhoeve AL, de Haes JC. Fatigue in cancer patients. Br J Cancer 1993; 68: 220-4

7   Smets EM, Visser MR, Willems-Groot AF, et al. Fatigue and radiotherapy: (A) experience in patients undergoing treatment. Br J Cancer 1998; 78: 899-906

8   Hickok JT, Morrow GR, McDonald S, Bellg AJ. Frequency and correlates of fatigue in lung cancer patients receiving radiation therapy: implications for management. J Pain Symptom Manage 1996; 11: 370-7

9   Richardson A. Measuring fatigue in patients with cancer. Support Care Cancer 1998; 6: 94-100

10   Smets EM, Garssen B, Cull A, de Haes JC. Application of the multidimensional fatigue inventory (MFI-20) in cancer patients receiving radiotherapy. Br J Cancer 1996; 73: 241-5

11   Greenberg DB, Sawicka J, Eisenthal S, Ross D. Fatigue syndrome due to localized radiation. J Pain Symptom Manage 1992; 7: 38-45

12   Monga U, Kerrigan AJ, Thornby J, Monga TN. Prospective study of fatigue in localized prostate cancer patients undergoing radiotherapy. Radiat Oncol Investig 1999; 7: 178-85

13   Okuyama T, Akechi T, Kugaya A, et al. Factors correlated with fatigue in disease-free breast cancer patients: application of the Cancer Fatigue Scale. Support Care Cancer 2000; 8: 215-22

14   Irvine D, Vincent L, Graydon JE, Bubela N, Thompson L. The prevalence and corre-lates of fatigue in patients receiving treatment with chemotherapy and radiotherapy. A comparison with the fatigue experienced by healthy individuals. Cancer Nurs 1994; 17: 367-78

15   Schwartz AL, Nail LM, Chen S, et al. Fatigue patterns observed in patients receiving chemotherapy and radiotherapy. Cancer Invest 2000; 18: 11-9

16   Kiebert GM, Curran D, Aaronson NK, et al. Quality of life after radiation therapy of cerebral low-grade gliomas of the adult: results of a randomized phase III trial on dose response (EORTC trial 22844). EORTC Radiotherapy Co-operative Group. Eur J Cancer 1998; 34: 1902-9

17   Lovely MP, Miaskowski C, Dodd M. Relationship between fatigue and quality of life in patients with glioblastoma multiforme. Oncol Nurs Forum 1999; 26: 921-5

18   Beard CJ, Propert KJ, Riekert PP, et al. Complications after treatment with external-beam irradiation in early-stage prostate cancer patients: a prospective multiinstitu-tional outcomes study. J Clin Oncol 1997; 15: 223-9

19   Nemoto K, Yamada S, Takai Y, Ogawa Y, Kakuto Y, Ariga H. Radiation therapy for low-grade astrocytomas: survival and QOL. Nippon Igaku Hoshasen Gakkai Zasshi 1997; 57: 336-40 (in Japanese)

20   Taphoorn MJ, Schiphordt AK, Snoek FJ, et al. Cognitive functions and quality of life in patients with low-grade gliomas: the impact of radiotherapy. Ann Neurol 1994; 36: 48-54

21   Norum J, Wist EA. Quality of life in survivors of Hodgkin's disease. Qual Life Res 1996; 5: 367-74

22   Abrahamsen AF, Loge JH, Hannisdal E, Holte H, Kvaloy S. Socio-medical situation for long survivors of Hodgkin's disease: a survey of 459 patients treated at one institution. Eur J Cancer 1998; 34: 1865-70

23   Macquart-Moulin G, Viens P, Genre D, et al. Concomitant chemotherapy for patients with nonmetastatic breast carcinoma: side effects, quality of life, and organization. Cancer 1999; 85; 2190-9

24   Woo B, Dibble SL, Piper BF, Keating SB, Weiss MC. Differences in fatigue by treatment methods in women with breast cancer. Oncol Nurs Forum 1998; 25: 915-20

25 Decker TW, Cline-Elsen J, Gallagher M. Relaxation therapy as an adjunct in radiation oncology. J Clin Psychol 1992; 48: 388-93

26 Mock V, Dow KH, Meares CJ, et al. Effects of exercise on fatigue, Physical functioning, and emotional distress during radiation therapy for breast cancer. Oncol Nurs Forum 1997; 24: 991-1000

27 Graydon JE, Bubela N, Irvine D, Vincent L. Fatigue-reducing strategies used by patients receiving treatment for cancer. Cancer Nurs 1995; 18: 23-8

28 Forester B, Kornfeld DS, Fleiss JL, Thompson S. Group psychotherapy during radiotherapy: effects on emotional and physical distress. Am J Psychiatry 1993; 150: 1700-6

29 Lavey RS. Clinical trial experience using erythropoietin during radiation therapy. Strahlenther Onkol 1998; 174 (suppl 4): 24-30

30 Walker BL, Nail LM, Larsen L, Magill J, Schwartz A. Concerns, affect, and cognitive disruption following completion of radiation treatment for localized breast or prostate cancer. Oncol Nurs Forum 1996; 23: 1181-7

31 Faithfull S, Brada M. Somnolence syndrome in adults following cranial irradiation for primary brain tumours. Clin Oncol (R Coll Radiol) 1998; 10: 250-4

32 Armstrong CL, Corn BW, Ruffer JE, Pruitt AA, Mollman JE, Phillips PC. Radiotherapeutic effects on brain function: double dissociation of memory systems. Neuropsychiatry Neuropsychol Behav Neurol 2000; 13: 101-11

33 Glantz MJ, Choy H, Yee L. Prophylactic cranial irradiation in small cell lung cancer: rationale, results, and recommendations. Semin Oncol 1997; 24: 477-83

34 Kaasa S, Aass N, Mastekaasa A, Lund E, Fossa SD. Psychosocial well-being in testicular cancer patients. Eur J Cancer 1991; 27: 1091-5

35 Carlsson M, Strang P, Bjurstrom C. Treatment modality affects long-term quality of life in gynaecological cancer. Anticancer Res 2000; 20: 563-8

36 Fieler VK. Side effects and quality of life in patients receiving high-dose rate brachytherapy. Oncol Nurs Forum 1997; 24: 545-53

37 Bye A, Ose T, Kaasa S. Quality of life during pelvic radiotherapy. Acta Obstet Gynecol Scand 1995; 74: 147-52

38 Ooi BS, Tjandra JJ, Green MD. Morbidities of adjuvant chemotherapy and radiotherapy for resectable rectal cancer: an overview. Dis Colon Rectum 1999; 42: 403-18

39 Turner S, Maher EJ, Young T, Young J, Vaughan Hudson G. What are the information priorities for cancer patients involved in treatment decisions? An experienced surrogate study in Hodgkin's disease. Br J Cancer 1996; 73: 222-7

40 de Graeff A, de Leeuw RJ, Ros WJ, et al. A prospective study on quality of life of laryngeal cancer patients treated with radiotherapy. Head Neck 1999; 21: 291-6

41 de Graeff A, de Leeuw JR, Ros WJ, Hordijk GJ, Blijham GH, Winnbust JA. A prospective study on quality of life of patients with cancer of the oral cavity or oropharynx treated with surgery with or without radiotherapy. Oral Oncol 1999; 35: 27-32

42 Lutz ST, Huang DT, Ferguson CL, Kavanagh BD, Tereilla OF, Lu J. A retrospective quality of life analysis using the Lung Cancer Symptom Scale in patients treated with palliative radiotherapy for advanced nonsmall cell lung cancer. Int J Radiat Oncol Biol Phys 1997; 37: 117-22

43 Langendijk JA, ten Velde GP, Aaronson NK, de Jong JM, Muller MJ, Wounters EF. Quality of life after palliative radiotherapy in non-small cell lung cancer: a prospective study. Int J Radiat Oncol Biol Phys 2000; 47: 149-55

44 Miaskowski C, Lee KA. Pain, fatigue, and sleep disturbances in oncology outpatients receiving radiation therapy for bone metastasis: a pilot study. J Pain Symptom Manage 1999; 17: 320-32

45 Altman GB, Lee CA. Strontium-89 for treatment of painful bone metastasis from prostate cancer. Oncol Nurs Forum 1996; 23: 523-7

ESO Scientific Updates, Vol. 5
Fatigue and Cancer
M. Marty and S. Pecorelli, editors

79

Approaches to Understanding the Mechanisms Involved in Fatigue Associated with Cancer and its Treatments: A Speculative Review

Paul L.R. Andrews[1] and Gary R. Morrow[2]

1   Department of Physiology, St George's Hospital Medical School, London, UK
2   University of Rochester Cancer Center, Rochester, NY, USA

Introduction

The inclusion of the word "speculative" in the title of this review reflects the current state of knowledge of the mechanism(s) responsible for the fatigue associated with cancer and its treatment. In many aspects our knowledge of fatigue mechanisms in cancer patients is at a similar stage to that at which our understanding of anticancer therapy-induced nausea and vomiting was about 20 years ago. At that time preclinical studies had identified the basic pathways by which nausea and vomiting could be induced by motion (vestibular system), by centrally acting drugs such as opiates (area postrema, also known as the "chemoreceptor trigger zone for vomiting") and gut stimulation (abdominal vagal afferents). However, little was known as to exactly which pathways were involved in emesis induced by anticancer therapies or how the pathways were activated by these stimuli, and as a result treatment was suboptimal. In the past 20 years this situation has changed dramatically with the recognition of the important role of the abdominal vagal afferents, a reassessment of the role of the area postrema, and the identification of the pivotal role of 5-hydroxytryptamine (5-HT) and 5-hydroxytryptamine-3 receptors (5-HT_3). The latter led to the use of potent, selective 5-HT_3 receptor antagonists (e.g. granisetron, ondansetron, tropisetron) to treat acute emesis induced by anticancer therapies [1,2]. Although these agents have revolutionised the treatment of anticancer therapy-induced emesis, they do not totally block nausea and vomiting in all patients in the acute phase and have little – if any – effect in the delayed phase; hence research continues and preclinical studies have identified a new class of antiemetic agents, the neurokinin-1 receptor antagonists, which appear

Address for correspondence: P. Andrews, Department of Physiology, St George's Hospital Medical School, Cranmer Terrace, London SW17 0RE, United Kingdom.
Tel.: +44-181-7255369, fax: +44-181-7252993, e-mail: pandrews@sghms.ac.uk

to be very broad spectrum agents as they can block emesis induced by stimuli acting on the gut, vestibular system or the area postrema. Translation of these results to humans has proven difficult but the results indicate that the identification of a "universal" antiemetic is no longer a theoretical possibility [3].

With regard to fatigue, we know a wide range of stimuli that can cause it, ranging from normal activities (e.g. exercise) to diseases (e.g. polio, myasthenia gravis), infections (e.g. influenza) and therapies (e.g. radiation). If the neuromuscular apparatus is compromised (e.g. myasthenia gravis, multiple sclerosis), it is not surprising that fatigue and weakness result [4]. For exercise, although intuitively one thinks that the source of the weakness is the muscles, there is a considerable body of evidence to implicate the central nervous system in aspects of exercise-induced fatigue [5]. What is now needed is that we look at the fatigue associated with cancer and its therapy in the light of the knowledge of the pathways identified for other forms of fatigue. An important insight into chemotherapy-induced emesis came from a careful pharmacological assessment of the results of clinical trials (e.g. high-dose metoclopramide). Although trials of pharmacological agents in fatigue syndromes are in their infancy, there are several indications that this may provide a useful source of information to guide mechanistic studies.

A survey by Coates almost 20 years ago [6] revealed that nausea and vomiting were regarded by patients undergoing chemotherapy as the side effects of most concern. Because of the introduction of effective antiemetic agents and the optimisation of therapeutic regimes, fatigue has now moved up such lists and this should be a major impetus to research. The quote below from Beard over 100 years ago on subjective states is often used in relation to fatigue but in a truncated form:

> Neurasthenia (nervous exhaustion) has been the central Africa of medicine – an unexplored territory into which few may enter and those few have been compelled to bring back reports that have been neither credited or comprehended.

The rapidly growing recognition of fatigue as a serious clinical problem with identifiable underlying mechanisms that are likely to be amenable to therapeutic interventions (including drugs) encourages the view that the above quote is no longer an accurate summary of the state of knowledge.

Is fatigue an appropriate biological response to cancer and its treatment?

The perhaps surprising answer to this question is arguably "yes" and leads to a subsidiary related question, "What is the function of fatigue?". If the feeling or sensation of fatigue has a function, it probably has at least two related roles: firstly, the sensation may be used as an indication that the activity being undertaken may lead to damage if continued and clearly this is analogous to the function of somatic pain in helping animals avoid physical damage; secondly, the sensation of fatigue or simply the genesis of weakness in limbs may be an important means by which an animal exposed to an "insult" will reduce its activity and perhaps be encouraged to seek refuge, the advantage of this being that the animal will have the opportunity to recover in relative safety. It is clearly not possible to test such teleological hypotheses, but anyone who has had influenza will recall how difficult it is to work; imagine if you were in the same situation and had to forage or hunt for your food whilst ensuring that you do not become food yourself!

Fatigue can be viewed as one component of the body's response to a toxic insult. In the natural world these toxins are frequently ingested agents and three main types of response are evoked:

i)   responses to deal with the toxin and to reduce its immediate impact – most notably vomiting and diarrhoea to "purge" the system but in addition there are systemic responses, such as fever [7] and a reduction in free plasma iron [8], which are also part of the host's defensive response [9];
ii)   nausea and other aversive responses to help the animal learn from the experience and avoid a similar problem in the future;
iii) fatigue and increased sleep to help the animal recover.

Clearly, in the natural world these responses are "appropriate", but how appropriate are they when encountered clinically? It appears that cancer and aspects of its treatment can activate several components of the above defensive system. Nausea, vomiting and diarrhoea are all inappropriate responses to cancer and its treatment as they do not help remove the causal agent and it is clear that they should be prevented if possible. This is particularly the case for nausea, which is one of the main factors in the genesis of anticipatory emetic responses. Fatigue is a far more complex issue. It can be argued that the fatigue would be an appropriate response to cancer itself in a similar way as it is considered to be for infection, especially bearing in mind that it is only in a very small fraction of a single percent of our evolutionary history that we have attempted to intervene in the natural course of cancer or infection. A potential conflict arises when one considers the fatigue induced by anticancer therapies rather than the cancer itself: on the one hand, as the fatigue has a considerable negative impact on the patient's quality of life (QOL) and his or her family, it should be regarded – like the emesis induced by anticancer therapies – as an undesirable "side effect" and hence be treated; on the other hand, as the treatment is inducing behavioural and systemic responses similar to those evoked by an infection and such responses are clearly part of the recovery process, perhaps they should not be treated.

These issues require debate. Perhaps consideration should be given to ways of uncoupling the subjective sensations (e.g. weakness, lack of motivation and feelings of overwhelming tiredness) responsible for the reduction in QOL from the systemic responses, and of classifying the systemic responses into those which may be aiding recovery (e.g. increased cytokines?) and those exacerbating the fatigue (e.g. anaemia?).

How can the mechanism of fatigue be identified?

The identification of the mechanism(s) of fatigue associated with cancer and its treatment will require a combination of animal and clinical studies. At present relatively few studies have investigated the problem directly and therefore most insights have come by comparison of cancer-related fatigue with that occurring in other situations, particularly exercise and chronic fatigue syndrome (CFS). Studies in humans have the advantage that questionnaires can be used and the patients asked to comment directly upon their symptoms. However, they are limited in the extent to which mechanisms may be studied. Thus both types of study are needed and must inform each other.

Human studies

Whilst studies with questionnaires have characterised the phenomenon of fatigue (however defined) [e.g. 10], it is important that such studies are now supplemented by the measurement of a range of physiological and biochemical parameters. For example, preliminary studies of gross locomotor activity using an Actigraph attached to the wrist have quantified the disruption of sleep patterns following radiotherapy [11]. In patients with advanced cancer, dynamometers have been used to show a reduction in hand grip strength [12]. Such measures of somatic activity provide a useful adjunct to the questionnaires in widespread use and will help to identify the relationships between the two parameters. Additionally, they will provide another dimension to interpreting results from therapeutic interventions that should help to identify mechanisms. Novel methods are needed for monitoring the activity of patients non-invasively in a home environment. Also, several of the studies that have been undertaken in patients with chronic fatigue syndrome and identified physiological changes (e.g. heightened prolactin response to d-fenfluramine [13]) need to be performed in patients with cancer to give insights into the applicability of research into CFS to cancer-related fatigue.

There is a growing body of information on chemical changes in the plasma of patients with cancer, with particular attention focused on the cytokines (e.g. TNF). Whilst such studies are useful in plotting the gross changes occurring, it is highly unlikely that they will identify a single systemic agent ("fatigue factor") that is responsible. There are several reasons for this (depressing?) conclusion: correlation between plasma levels and a tissue response is always problematic as the secretion of the responsible factor may be episodic and, unless sampling frequency is very high over a prolonged period, this may be missed; and the plasma may not be the compartment of interest. For example, it is widely accepted that 5-hydroxytryptamine (5-HT) plays a major role in the acute phase of emesis induced by anticancer therapies, but the key site is within the wall of the gut in the basal region of the enterochromaffin cells – plasma levels of 5-HT do not rise [14]. Thus, although there may be a measurable change in a transmitter or modulator, it may occur in a compartment not readily measurable such as the brain or the cerebrospinal fluid; it has been known for 20 years that plasma antidiuretic hormone (ADH, vasopressin) is massively increased in subjects experiencing nausea caused by diverse stimuli (e.g. cytotoxic drugs, motion, pregnancy) [15]. Similar increases in ADH have been measured in animals and injection of ADH can induce nausea. Despite this body of evidence (and an equally impressive one concerning gastric rhythms and nausea) we still do not know whether the ADH increase is a cause or effect.

The above does not suggest that the measurements should not be made but that the results should be interpreted with considerable caution and particularly that, even if a correlation is found, this is a long way from showing causality.

Animal studies

Animal studies of fatigue mechanisms are in their infancy, probably because fatigue has only relatively recently been recognised as a serious and potentially treatable condition in humans. Studying fatigue in animals entails many of the same problems as studying nausea, particularly that of demonstrating that what is observed in animals equates to the human situation. The advantage of animal studies is that fundamental mechanisms can be more readily studied and pharmacological interventions investigated.

A study of the "sickness behaviours" (including fatigue, anorexia, malaise, listlessness and inability to concentrate) associated with cholestatic liver disease serves to illustrate the type of animal study which has been undertaken to model human disease in which fatigue may be the presenting symptom [16]. In rats, bile duct resection was used to mimic cholestatic disease [17]. This procedure resulted in reduced activity in an open field (a measure of exploratory activity in a stressful environment) associated with a blunted plasma adrenocorticotrophic hormone (ACTH) response, low basal hypothalamic corticotrophin releasing hormone (CRH) levels, and a blunted CRH response to restraint stress. This suggests that some of the behavioural effects of cholestatic disease are caused by damage to the hypothalamic-pituitary-adrenal axis (HPA), which has frequently been implicated in the chronic fatigue syndrome (see below). The authors speculated that the central endocrine changes may be mediated by cytokines, as elevated plasma levels of IL-6 and TNF-alpha have been measured in bile duct resected mice, and this is supported by studies in humans with primary biliary cirrhosis. A recent case report recorded relief from fatigue using the 5-HT$_3$ receptor antagonist ondansetron in a patient with chronic liver disease [18]. If this observation is substantiated then the rat model of bile duct resection may provide a valuable tool in which the role of 5-HT and the HPA in the genesis of fatigue and related symptoms can be investigated.

Testable hypotheses

In the section below a number of hypotheses are outlined to illustrate how muscle activity or the drive to undertake such activity may be reduced by cancer and its treatment. What we are unable to say is where the sensation of fatigue or lack of energy is perceived and in this sense fatigue again has parallels with nausea. Additionally, the initiating mechanism(s) is far from clear. For example, a fundamental issue is how much the fatigue is due to the tumour, how much to the treatment, and how much to other effects or their indirect consequences (e.g. deconditioning, cachexia, depression). It is clear that fatigue can be evoked by illnesses other than cancer (e.g. influenza), so it is likely that the mechanism is not unique to cancer but cancer is one of the many ways in which this response can be induced. Again, this is analogous to nausea and vomiting: there are multiple ways by which they can be evoked but all converge on a common output. The contribution of therapy as opposed to cancer is very hard to assess, as patients are not usually studied both before and during therapy. The impression gained from the literature is that the therapy is the factor which makes the major contribution to fatigue but it must be emphasised that this needs to be investigated objectively. Studies of the victims of accidental irradiation have shown that these subjects suffer from fatigue in addition to the other side effects associated with radiotherapy [19]. Thus the presence of a tumour is not essential for the induction of fatigue, although a tumour or other factors (e.g. surgery) may potentiate the effect. It would be of considerable interest to know whether patients who receive chemotherapy in error experience fatigue.

It must be emphasised that, with the exception of anaemia, the vast majority of information presented below is derived from the study of fatigue in settings other than cancer and, whilst such models may apply to cancer fatigue, their applicability requires formal testing. Irrespective of this we believe that these models provide useful approaches to the problem.

Altered muscle metabolism

The skeletal muscles have not surprisingly been the predominant focus of mechanistic studies of exercise-induced fatigue and have revealed the complexity of understanding the processes underlying muscle fatigue defined as "any exercise-induced reduction in the ability to exert muscle force or power, regardless of whether or not the task can be sustained" [5]. The fundamental mechanism of force generation in skeletal muscle is the interaction between actin filaments and myosin cross-bridges; factors which interfere with this interaction will lead to a reduction in force, i.e., fatigue. Focusing on factors in the muscle, Ca^{++}, K^+, H^+, Pi, ADP and ATP are all able to directly or indirectly influence the actin-myosin interaction and hence force generation. It is therefore possible that cancer or its treatment could produce fatigue by modulation of any of these factors. In studies of CFS there is no consistent evidence that the problem resides in the periphery, i.e., the muscle or its innervation [20]. Although an involvement of the skeletal muscle or its direct innervation has not been excluded in cancer patients, it is essential that studies investigating this problem include measurements of both voluntary muscle contraction and that evoked by electrical stimulation of the nerve supplying the same muscles ("twitch interpolation") [5]. This is one of the important techniques which allows a distinction to be made between central mechanisms (brain and spinal cord) and those operating at the level of the neuromuscular system.

A recent study in patients with CFS did provide some evidence for a defect in adenosine triphosphate (ATP) metabolism. Adenosine triphosphate is the major source of energy via the splitting of high-energy phosphate bonds for a range of cellular processes including those responsible for the generation of mechanical work (contraction) in skeletal muscle. Thus, it is self-evident that depletion of ATP would compromise the ability to do mechanical work.

Normally, ATP can be quickly replenished with most cellular ATP being formed in mitochondria by oxidative phosphorylation. In a study of patients with chronic fatigue syndrome, increased 2'-5' A synthetase and RNAase L activity led to depleted cellular ATP which was thought to be "a pivotal lesion responsible for severe fatigue, cognitive difficulties or other disturbances" [21]. Other investigators have also found impaired synthesis of ATP and defective muscle energy metabolism together with impaired voluntary activation of skeletal muscle during sustained intense exercise in a proportion of patients with CFS [22]. In non-dialysed patients with chronic renal failure who often complain of muscle weakness and fatigue after minor physical activity and may suffer from myopathy related to uraemia, muscle biopsies showed significantly low ATP and creatine phosphate levels [23].

Nicotinamide adenine dinucleotide (NAD) is a key coenzyme in the process of oxidative phosphorylation and is therefore important in the formation of ATP [23]. In a randomised, double-blind crossover study the ability of oral NADH, the reduced form of the coenzyme NAD which is used to ameliorate symptoms of CFS including fatigue, cognitive dysfunction and sleep disturbance, was compared to placebo. Eight of 26 patients (31%) showed at least 10% improvement in their score on a questionnaire measuring fatigue, memory, ability to concentrate, sleep disturbance and mood, and reported decreased fatigue, decreased symptoms overall and improved quality of life taking the study drug compared to 2/26 (8%) taking placebo (p<0.05) [21]. A similar study would be worth undertaking in patients with cancer but should include objective measurements of muscle function.

Anaemia

Fatigue and dyspnoea have long been known to be associated with anaemia, and anaemia can occur in patients with cancer and be exacerbated by many types of anticancer therapy via multiple mechanisms including TNF, IL-1 and IFN-gamma [24]. Although it would appear to be self-evident that anaemia causes fatigue and there is some evidence in patients undergoing chemotherapy that "energy" may be increased as the anaemia is treated with rHuEPO [25], the mechanism(s) linking the two are far from clear. Part of the reason may be the slow onset of the anaemia giving the patients' cardiorespiratory system time to adapt and enabling patients to reduce their physical demands, but this still leaves the nature of the mechanistic link open. Whilst hypoxia-related impairment of organ function is usually implicated as the causal mechanism [26] and there is no doubt that hypoxia can induce fatigue-like symptoms and dyspnoea, the extent to which this is the causal mechanism has not been investigated in cancer patients. If it is organ hypoxia, then which is the critical organ(s) or system(s) (e.g. brain, skeletal muscle)?

The reason for drawing attention to this is that anaemia can be induced in animal models by tumours and cytotoxic drugs and cancer-related anaemia responds to erythropoietin in animals. It is therefore possible to model quite accurately both the disease and its treatment in an animal model. In view of this it should be relatively easy to investigate in detail the mechanisms linking fatigue to anaemia induced by cancer and its treatment and perhaps provide more general insights into the pathophysiology of cancer-related fatigue.

Vagal afferent activation

Several experimental animal studies have demonstrated that skeletal muscle activity can be reflexly modulated by vagal afferents ("sensory" fibres). Particular attention has focused on pulmonary vagal afferents, although abdominal vagal afferents have been shown to have a similar effect. Activation of pulmonary vagal afferents by either electrical stimulation or a range of neuroactive chemicals (e.g. 5-hydroxytryptamine, nicotine, thromboxane A2 agonist) has been shown to reduce reflex activation of the knee-jerk reflex and locomotion in one study. A population of pulmonary receptors known as J-receptors have been implicated in the above responses. It has been proposed that the function of these afferents is to induce the sensation of breathlessness/dyspnoea associated with intense exercise and to limit the exercise to prevent tissue damage [27]. Evidence from humans supporting this hypothesis is scant, as would be expected, but in a patient with total blockage to the right lung who experienced dyspnoea, tachypnoea and excessive ventilation upon exercise it was shown that section of the right vagus not only relieved the dyspnoea but also increased the work tolerance of the patient [28]. It must be emphasised that the role of such receptors in humans and the effects they can mediate is still controversial [29], but in view of their possible involvement in both dyspnoea and muscle tone further studies to investigate their role in dyspnoea and fatigue associated with cancer are essential.

Although the focus has been on pulmonary afferents, abdominal vagal afferents have also been shown to be capable of modulating skeletal muscle activity in the rat [30]. Abdominal vagal afferents are known to be active following cytotoxic drug administration and radiation exposure, as they have been shown to be implicated in the emesis induced by these two types of therapy [31]. In addition, vagal afferents have been shown to respond to a variety of endogenous chemicals including 5-HT, substance P, prostaglandin and cytokines (e.g. IL-1B). 5-HT_3 receptor antagonists have been used to treat the acute emesis induced by anticancer chemotherapy for about 10 years. If 5-HT acting on vagal 5-HT_3 receptors is involved in fatigue, then perhaps it would have been expected that some evidence supporting this would have "emerged" from antiemetic studies. This does not appear to be the case but it must be borne in mind that, as an assessment of fatigue is rarely included in antiemetic studies, such information would only arise from patient self-reports. In addition, antiemetics are only given acutely but there may be a more chronic release of 5-HT involved in fatigue requiring long-term treatment with 5-HT_3 receptor antagonists. In preliminary studies granisetron has been reported to improve performance status in two patients treated with alpha-2b recombinant interferon [32] and ondansetron relieved fatigue in a patient with chronic liver disease [18]. These results are consistent with an involvement of 5-HT and 5-HT_3 receptors in the genesis of fatigue but further studies are needed. It is of interest that Novartis has filed a patent claim (WO 0037073) for the use of 5-HT_3 receptor antagonists to treat chronic fatigue syndrome. The above section has focused on peripheral 5-HT but this does not exclude a role for central 5-HT (see below).

In the context of cancer and its treatment it is being proposed that released chemicals (e.g. cytokines) cause a low-level activation and/or sensitisation of vagal afferents leading to a reflex reduction in the somatic motorneurone drive to the postural skeletal muscles. This reduction in drive may be perceived as an inability to complete a motor task or as a feeling that more effort (i.e. central motor drive) is required to complete the task than was usually required or was anticipated.

Cytokines and the abdominal vagal afferents are also perhaps of more general relevance to understanding the effects of cancer and its therapy on the body as a whole. In rats, both the vagus and cytokines have been implicated in the induction of "sickness syndrome": a syndrome induced by intraperitoneal injection of bacterial lipopolysaccharide or IL-1β characterised by an initial phase with hyperalgesia/allodynia, increased activity and fever and a later phase with hypoalgesia, decreased activity, increased sleep and either fever or hypothermia. Some aspects of this are resonant of the effects of cancer and its treatment. In the piglet, the emetic effects of intraperitoneal lipolysaccharide are abolished by cervical vagotomy and cyclooxygenase inhibitors but not by a 5-HT_3 receptor antagonist, implicating prostaglandins in vagal afferent activation [33]. In addition, in the rat intraperitoneal injection of IL-1β via abdominal vagal activation has been shown to increase induction of IL-1β mRNA in the brainstem (as would be expected because the vagal afferents terminate here), the hypothalamus and the hippocampus [34]. As the hypothalamus and higher regions of the brain have been implicated in the pathogenesis of fatigue, this pathway could provide a mechanism by which a stimulus with a primarily peripheral action could have an immediate "acute" effect via a reflex (e.g. a vagal reflex reduction in muscle tone via the brainstem) and a sustained "chronic" effect (the "footprint" of the treatment).

Central 5-HT dysregulation

Evidence implicating central 5-HT in the genesis of fatigue comes from two main sources: exercise physiology and pharmacological studies of patients with chronic fatigue syndrome.

Exercise physiology

A considerable body of evidence has implicated the brain in the mechanism of fatigue associated with exercise – the so-called "central fatigue" defined as "a progressive exercise-induced reduction in voluntary activation of muscle" [5]. Prolonged exercise is known to increase blood levels of tryptophan, the amino acid precursor of 5-HT, and as 5-HT is known to be involved in sleep, aggression and mood it was proposed that it could be mediating the mental fatigue occurring during and after heavy exercise [35]. The reason why central 5-HT levels could increase during exercise is because tryptophan and branch-chain amino acids enter the brain using the same carrier and thus can compete for transport. During exercise the plasma level of branch-chain amino acids decreases because the latter are taken up by the active muscle. This reduces competition with tryptophan for the carrier and allows more tryptophan access to the brain, possibly leading to an increase in 5-HT in specific brain regions. In rats, sustained exercise increased 5-HT levels in only two of six areas investigated, namely the hypothalamus and the brainstem [36], but administration of a 5-HT agonist to rats caused a dose-related decrease in running [37] and an antagonist improved performance [38]. Studies in healthy humans using ingestion of branch-chain amino acids to compete with tryptophan and hence prevent the presumed rise in central 5-HT during exercise have yielded promising results. For example, in subjects exercising on a bicycle ergometer at 70% of their VO_2 max for 60 min, ingestion of branch-chain amino acids reduced the subjects' ratings of perceived exertion and ratings of mental fatigue measured using two different Borg scales [39]. Post exercise there was an improvement in the score in Stroop's Colour Word Test. Interestingly, ingestion of branch-chain amino acids did not have a significant effect on the scores when subjects were exercising maximally. Some evidence has been presented suggesting that consumption of branch-chain amino acids may improve performance in slower but not faster marathon runners [35]. This latter observation is of particular interest as an indirect study of central sensitivity to 5-HT using prolactin secretion reported evidence for a reduced sensitivity in endurance-trained athletes compared to untrained subjects [40].

Further evidence linking central 5-HT to exercise endurance comes from studies of the effect of drugs in exercising subjects. A single 20 mg oral dose of paroxetine (an SSRI) reduced the time that subjects could exercise at 70% of VO_2 max on a bicycle ergometer [41] and the $5HT_{1A}$ receptor agonist buspirone had a similar effect during exercise at 80% VO_2 max and also increased the rating of perceived exhaustion [42].

Taken together, the above studies are consistent in providing evidence that an increase in central 5-HT at an as yet unidentified site in healthy individuals can increase the perception of exertion and in some cases reduce endurance.

Chronic fatigue syndrome

In patients with chronic fatigue syndrome there is some evidence for changes in central 5-HT or its receptors and these may be the cause of some of the hypothalamic-pituitary-adrenal axis dysfunction discussed below. As a number of pituitary hormones have their secretion influenced by 5-HT it is possible to probe some central serotonergic pathways by using the HPA response to 5-HT receptor agonists. Enhanced prolactin responses have been reported in patients with CFS, but not patients with primary depression, to buspirone (5-HT$_{1A}$ receptor agonist) and d-fenfluramine (5-HT$_2$ receptor agonist) [13,43-45]. Although there are several possible explanations for these results and the agonists used may not be as selective as originally thought, the results provide support for a hypersensitivity/upregulation of the central 5-HT receptors regulating prolactin secretion. Such studies provide a model for the type of study that needs to be undertaken in patients undergoing treatment for cancer.

To summarise the above studies: the sensations of fatigue associated with heavy exercise may be the result of an increased level of 5-HT in an as yet unidentified region of the brain; in chronic fatigue syndrome there is limited evidence for an increased sensitivity of the HPA to 5-HT. Taken together, these observations suggest that studies of central serotonergic function are urgently needed in patients undergoing treatment for cancer and these could take the form of using selective 5-HT receptor agonists, selective 5-HT receptor antagonists, SSRIs or modification of central 5-HT by means of dietary branch-chain amino acids.

Hypothalamic-pituitary axis dysfunction

The above studies suggesting dysfunction of central serotonergic pathways also provide evidence that there may be a dysfunction in the hypothalamic pituitary axis and the studies here should be considered together with those above. There are several examples of hypothalamic dysfunction in patients with chronic fatigue syndrome which provide pointers for studies in patients with cancer:

i)   in patients with postviral fatigue syndrome a lack of correlation was found between plasma osmolality and plasma levels of vasopressin (antidiuretic hormone), suggesting that either the hypothalamic osmoreceptors were damaged or there was a defect in the posterior pituitary [46]. This study is of particular interest because it investigated a hormone produced by the posterior pituitary whereas the anterior pituitary hormones have been the focus of all other studies;

ii) there is evidence for a central downregulation of the HPA axis in patients
    with chronic fatigue syndrome leading to mild hypocortisolism. The cause
    is most probably a defect in the corticotrophin-releasing hormone (CRH)
    neurones in the hypothalamus. In the section above on animal models, a re-
    duction in CRH was reported in a rat model of cholestatic disease giving
    rise to sickness syndrome. CRH is of particular interest because of its pivot-
    al role in the stress responses mediated by the HPA. The HPA studies in pa-
    tients with chronic fatigue syndrome contrast with those in patients with
    major depression who have evidence of central upregulation of the HPA and
    mild hypercortisolism [47-49].

Conclusions and questions

In this chapter we have attempted to look at cancer-related fatigue from a
novel perspective and have deliberately been speculative to provoke discussion
and research into mechanisms. Although many aspects of cancer-related fatigue
have been characterised, perhaps with the exception of anaemia, there has
been relatively little research into its mechanisms in contrast to fatigue induced
either by exercise or chronic fatigue syndrome. It is clear from recent surveys
both in the US and the UK that fatigue has become the problem of most concern
to patients, supplanting nausea and vomiting, which can now be alleviated –
although not completely prevented – by drugs. We believe that for cancer-related fatigue research a similar combination of circumstances now exists to that
which existed for emesis induced by anticancer therapies in the early 1980s: a
serious problem with an impact on QOL for patients and carers; greater recognition of the problem by nurses than doctors; limited methodologies for study,
particularly of the subjective components (i.e. nausea); clinical trials suggestive
of therapeutic approaches; mechanistic data from human studies of analogous
clinical problems; potentially relevant animal models; a growing recognition by
the pharmaceutical industry that there is a "target" for drug discovery.

Taking an overview we draw the following conclusions and make a number of
comments:

- Fatigue is a relevant biological response ("physiological coping strategy")
  to cancer and its therapy and explaining this to patients may help them better understand what is happening and perhaps improve their ability to cope
  and enhance the efficacy of any management strategies.
- The main factor inducing fatigue is the therapy itself, although the mecha-
  nism(s) by which this is mediated are far from clear. Cytokines appear to be
  the most likely candidates to initiate the response, but how this is translated into the subjective and objective components of fatigue is not known.
  The role of other factors such as surgery and the way in which they may in-
  teract with or potentiate the primary mechanisms must not be overlooked.
- Several mechanisms have been reviewed, all of which can be tested and as a
  result rejected, helping to narrow the list of possible mechanisms. In particu-

lar, investigation of the central changes associated with exercise and chronic fatigue syndrome need to be studied in patients with cancer-related fatigue to see whether these situations could provide models for cancer-related fatigue. Non-invasive techniques such as magnetic stimulation [29] have proven invaluable for studying the cortical control of motor pathways and, in conjunction with other techniques, for helping differentiate central and peripheral fatigue mechanisms. Similar studies could be undertaken in small groups of patients with cancer-related fatigue.

• Although it is possible that studies (particularly of pharmacological therapies) in cancer patients may provide important insights into the mechanism(s) responsible for cancer-related fatigue, the contribution of preclinical studies should not be neglected. Animal models of chronic fatigue syndromes are poorly developed, although studies of cholestasis suggest that animal models have features in common with the patient. Models already exist to study the effects of a tumour (particularly breast or testicular) and the effects of chemotherapy, but they have not been combined with the intention of investigating fatigue mechanisms. The development of appropriate animal models would expedite understanding of the mechanism(s) and also provide a model in which to investigate novel therapies. One of the major mechanistic challenges is to understand why in many cases the fatigue is so prolonged. We would argue from this that prophylaxis would be a more realistic target for pharmacological therapy rather than attempting to treat fatigue once established. This approach does not exclude treatment of factors which may contribute to cancer-related fatigue, such as anaemia and cachexia.

References

1   Sanger GJ, Andrews PLR. Emesis. In: Farthing MJG, Ballinger AB, eds. Drug therapy for gastrointestinal and liver disease. Martin Dunitz Publ, 2001 (in press)

2   Morrow GR, Hickok JT, Rosenthal SN. Progress in reducing nausea and emesis. Comparisons of ondansetron (Zofran), granisetron (Kytril), and tropisetron (Navoban). Cancer 1995; 76: 343-57

3   Andrews PLR. Postoperative nausea and vomiting. In: Herbert MK, Holzer P, Roewer N, eds. Problems of the gastrointestinal tract in anesthesia, the perioperative period, and intensive care. Berlin, Heidelberg: Springer-Verlag, 1999; 267-88

4   McComas AJ, Miller RG, Gandevia SC. Fatigue brought on by malfunction of the central and peripheral nervous systems. In: Gandevia SC, Enoka RM, McComas AJ, Stuart DG, Thomas CK, eds. Fatigue. Neural and muscular mechanisms. New York: Plenum Press, 1995; 495-512

5   Gandevia SC, Allen GM, McKenzie DK. Central fatigue. Critical issues, quantification and practical implications. In: Gandevia SC, Enoka RM, McComas AJ, Stuart DG, Thomas CK, eds. Fatigue. Neural and muscular mechanisms. New York: Plenum Press, 1995; 281-94

6   Coates A, Abraham S, Kaye SB, et al. On the receiving end – patient perception of the side effects of cancer chemotherapy. Eur J Cancer Clin Oncol 1983; 19: 203-8

7   Kluger MJ. Fever: role of pyrogens and cryogens. Physiol Rev 1991; 71: 93-127

8   Weinberg ED. Iron withholding: a defence against infection and neoplasia. Physiol Rev 1984; 64: 65-102

9   Long NC. Evolution of infectious disease: How evolutionary forces shape physiological responses to pathogens. News Physiol Sci 1996; 11: 83-90

10   Hickok JT, Morrow GR, McDonald S, Bellq AJ. Frequency and correlates of fatigue in lung cancer patients receiving radiation therapy: Implications for management. J Pain Symptom Manage 1996; 11: 370-7

11   Hickok JT, Roscoe JA, Morrow GR, Bushunow P. Wrist actigraphy as a measure of fatigue. Proc Am Soc Clin Oncol 1998; 17: 60a

12   Stone P, Hardy J, Broadley K, Tookman AJ, Kurowska A, Hern RA. Fatigue in advanced cancer: a prospective controlled cross-sectional study. Br J Cancer 1999; 79: 1479-86

13   Cleare A, Bearn J, Allain T. Contrasting neuroendocrine responses in depression and chronic fatigue syndrome. J Affect Disord 1995; 35: 283-9

14   Andrews PLR. 5-HT$_3$ receptor antagonists and antiemesis. In: King FD, Jones BJ, Sanger GJ, eds. 5-hydroxytryptamine-3 receptor antagonists. Boca Raton, USA: CRC Press, Inc, 1994; 255-317

15   Koch KL. A noxious trio: nausea, gastric dysrhythmias and vasopressin. Neurogast Motil 1997; 9: 141-2

16   Vierling JM. Primary biliary cirrhosis. In: Zakim D, Boyer TD, eds. Hepatology: a textbook of liver disease, Vol 2, Ed 2. Philadelphia: Saunders, 1990; 1161-3

17   Swain MG, Maric M. Defective corticotropin-releasing hormone mediated neuroendocrine and behavioral responses in cholestatic rats: Implications for cholestatic liver disease-related sickness behaviors. Hepatology 1995; 22: 1560-4

18   Jones EA. Relief from profound fatigue associated with chronic liver disease by long-term ondansetron therapy. The Lancet 1999; 354: 397

19   Anno GH, Baum SJ, Withers HR, Young RW. Symptomatology of acute radiation effects in humans after exposure to doses of 0.5-30 Gy. Health Phys 1989; 56: 821-38

20   Wessely S, Hotopf M, Sharpe M, eds. Chronic fatigue and its syndromes. Oxford: Oxford University Press, 1998; 428

21   Forsyth LM, Preuss HG, MacDowell AL, Chiazze L, Birkmayer GD, Bellanti JA. Therapeutic effects of oral NADH on the symptoms of patients with chronic fatigue syndrome. Ann Allerg Asthma Immunol 1999; 82: 185-91

22   Lane RJ, Barrett MC, Taylor DJ, Kemp GJ, Lodi R. Heterogeneity in chronic fatigue syndrome: evidence from magnetic resonance spectroscopy of muscle. Neuromuscul Disord 1998; 8: 204-9

23   Pastoris O, Aquilina R, Foppa P, et al. Altered muscle energy metabolism in post-absorptive patients with chronic renal failure. Scand J Urol Nephrol 1997; 31: 281-7

24   Groopman JE, Itri LM. Chemotherapy-induced anaemia in adults: Incidence and treatment. J Natl Cancer Inst 1999; 91: 1616-35

25   Demetri GD, Kris M, Wade J, Degos L, Cella D. Quality-of-life benefit in chemotherapy patients treated with epoetin alfa is independent of disease response or tumor type: Results from a prospective community oncology study. J Clin Oncol 1998; 16: 3412-25

26   Mercuriali F, Inghilleri G. Treatment of anemia in cancer patients: transfusion or rHu-EPO. This volume of the European School of Oncology Scientific Update Series

27   Paintal AS. Sensations from J receptors. News Physiol 1995; 10: 238-43

28   Davies SF, McQuaid KR, Iber C, et al. Extreme dyspnea from unilateral pulmonary venous obstruction. Demonstration of a vagal mechanism and relief by right vagotomy. Am Rev Respir Dis 1987; 136: 184-8

29   Gandevia SC, Butler JE, Taylor JL, Crawford MR. Absence of viscerosomatic inhibition with injections of lobeline designed to activate human pulmonary C fibres. J Physiol 1998; 511: 289-300

30   Kawaski K, Kodama M, Matsushita A. Caerulein, a cholecystokinin-related peptide, depresses somatic function via the vagal afferent system. Life Sci 1983; 33: 1045-50

31 Andrews PLR, Davis CJ. The physiology of emesis induced by anti-cancer therapy. In: Reynolds DJM, Andrews PLR, Davis CJ, eds. Serotonin and the scientific basis of anti-emetic therapy. Oxford Clin Commun 1995; 25-49

32 Drapkin R, Barolo JL, Blower PR. Effect of granisetron on performance status during high-dose interferon therapy. Oncology 1999; 57: 303-5

33 Girod V, Bouvier M, Grelot L. Characterization of lipopolysaccharide-induced emesis in conscious piglets: effects of cervical vagotomy, cyclooxygenase inhibitors and a 5-HT3 receptor antagonist. Neuropharmacol 2000; 39: 2329-35

34 Hansen MK, Taishi P, Chen Z, Krueger JM. Vagotomy blocks the induction of inter-leukin-1β (IL-1β) mRNA in the brain of rats in response to systemic IL-1β. J Neurosci 1998; 18: 2247-53

35 Newsholme EA, Blomstrand E. Tryptophan, 5-hydroxytryptamine and a possible explanation for central fatigue. In: Gandevia SC, Enoka RM, McComas AJ, Stuart DG, Thomas CK, eds. Fatigue. Neural and muscular mechanisms. New York: Plenum Press, 1995; 315-20

36 Bloomstrand E, Perrett D, Parry-Billings M, Newsholme EA. Effect of sustained exer-cise on plasma amino acid concentrations and on 5-hydroxytryptamine metabolism in six different brain regions of the rat. Acta Physiol Scand 1989; 136: 473-81

37 Bailey SP, Davis JM, Ahlborn EN. Effect of increased brain serotonergic activity on endurance performance in the rat. Acta Physiol Scand 1992; 145: 75-6

38 Bailey SP, Davis JM, Ahlborn EN. Neuroendocrine and substrate responses to altered brain 5-HT activity during prolonged exercise to fatigue. J Appl Physiol 1993; 74: 3006-12

39 Blomstrand E, Hassmen P, Ekblom B, Newsholme EA. Influence of ingesting a solution of branched-chain amino acids on perceived exertion during exercise. Acta Physiol Scand 1997; 159: 41-9

40 Jakeman PM, Hawthorne JE, Maxwell SRJ, Kendall MJ, Holder G. Evidence for down-regulation of hypothalamic 5-hydroxytryptamine receptor function in endurance-trained athletes. Exp Physiol 1994; 79: 461-4

41 Wilson WM, Maughan RJ. Evidence for a possible role of 5-hydroxytryptamine in the genesis of fatigue in man: Administration of paroxetine, a 5-HT re-uptake inhibitor, re-duces the capacity to perform prolonged exercise. Exp Physiol 1992; 77: 921-4

42 Marvin G, Sharma A, Aston W, Field C, Kendall MJ, Jones DA. The effects of buspirone on perceived exertion and time to fatigue in man. Exp Physiol 1997; 82: 1057-60

43 Bakheit A, Behan P, Dinan T, Gray C, O'Keane V. Possible upregulation of hypo-thalamic 5-hydroxytryptamine receptors in patients with postviral fatigue syndrome. Br Med J 1992; 304: 1010-2

44 Sharpe M, Clements A, Hawton P, Young A, Sargent P, Cowen P. Increased prolactin re-sponse to buspirone in chronic fatigue syndrome. J Affect Disord 1996; 41: 71-6

45 Sharpe M, Hawton K, Clements A, Cowen P. Increased brain serotonin function in men with chronic fatigue syndrome. Br Med J 1997; 315: 164-5

46 Bakheit AMO, Behan PO, Watson WS. Abnormal arginine-vasopressin secretion and water metabolism in patients with postviral fatigue syndrome. Acta Neurol Scand 1993; 87: 234-8

47 Demitrack MA. Neuroendocrine aspects of chronic fatigue syndrome: A commentary. Am J Med 1998; 105: 11S-14S

48 Demitrack MA, Dale JK, Straus SE, et al. Evidence for impaired activation of the hypo-thalamic-pituitary-adrenal axis in patients with chronic fatigue syndrome. J Clin En-docrin Metab 1991; 73: 1224-34

49 Komaroff AL, Buchwald DS. Chronic fatigue syndrome: An update. Ann Rev Med 1998; 49: 1-13

ESO Scientific Updates, Vol. 5
Fatigue and Cancer
M. Marty and S. Pecorelli, editors
© 2001 Elsevier Science B.V. All rights reserved

Definition of Fatigue, Diagnostic Criteria, and Algorithms of Patient Evaluation

Karin Magnusson

Department of Oncology, Unit of Research and Development, Sahlgrenska University Hospital, Göteborg, Sweden

Introduction

The definition of a term is complicated when we consider all the different nuances of meaning in different languages and cultures. In the English and French languages, the word fatigue is used to express feelings of extreme, unusual tiredness, in other languages the term fatigue does not exist [1]. Fatigue is a difficult phenomenon to define and many of the existing definitions incorporate notions of a subjective experience [2].

Fatigue is a word that is not only used in the contexts of medicine, nursing, and psychology but also, for example, in the technical area of engineering [1]. Fatigue may describe a number of experiences, from the exhaustion a healthy individual may feel after running a marathon, to the sleepiness a person experiences after having been awake for a long time, to the experience of extreme, unusual tiredness an individual with a severe disease may feel.

Fatigue is a common feeling, experienced daily by most people as a state of increased discomfort and decreased ability to function [3]. Fatigue occurs as a symptom in almost every medical and psychiatric condition, as well as being a common reaction to nonpathological physical and psychological strain and stress. Fatigue seems to be used as an umbrella term to describe a variety of sensations or feelings and a variety of expressions of decreased capacity at physical, mental, psychological, or social levels [1]. In epidemiological studies among the general population, 20% reported substantial fatigue [4]. We now know that, depending on the individual situation and the specific disease and treatment, among other factors, the reporting percentage is much higher among cancer patients.

The meaning of fatigue is unclear. In healthy individuals fatigue might serve as a protective and/or pleasant response to physical or psychological

---

Address for correspondence: K. Magnusson, Department of Oncology, Unit of Research and Development, Sahlgrenska University Hospital, 413 45 Göteborg, Sweden. Tel.: +46-31-3424013; e-mail: karin.magnusson@oncology.gu.se

stress. Conversely, for patients with a chronic disease it may become a major distressing symptom [5]. For cancer patients fatigue is a concern at many points during the disease process, and the problem is not easily resolved.

In a study by Magnusson et al. [6] all respondents stated that the fatigue they experienced in connection with their disease was totally different from the fatigue they had experienced as healthy individuals. Glaus et al. [7], in a study exploring the concept of fatigue in cancer patients and healthy individuals, showed that there was a difference between cancer patients and healthy individuals in the characteristics of their experience of fatigue/tiredness. For both groups the physical sensations of fatigue were dominant, compared with affective and cognitive sensations. However, whereas in healthy individuals tiredness is experienced as a circadian phenomenon indicated by limbs feeling heavy from daily activity and by a sensation of sleepiness after work, the cancer patients' experience encompasses decreased physical performance, feeling unusually and extremely tired or weak, and needing more rest [1]. A major difference between fatigue in healthy individuals and in illness is that fatigue occurs as a negative symptom of the illness and often does not disappear after rest [8].

Fatigue has been studied in connection with situations other than cancer, e.g. childbearing, chronic heart failure, chronic fatigue syndrome (CFS), and multiple sclerosis (MS), and in healthy individuals. It looks like fatigue is a universal complaint that may or may not be related to medical diagnosis or result from therapeutic treatment. A review of studies of fatigue among different populations makes it clear that fatigue is a nonspecific phenomenon, related to different medical diagnoses, in particular chronic diseases and their treatments [9]. A literature search by Milligan and Pugh [10] concluded that fatigue has four dimensions: a) physiological, b) psychological, c) situational, and d) performance. The experience and definition of fatigue in other groups studied are similar to those in cancer patients.

Studies have documented that patients with MS [11,12] and patients with cancer [5] report more fatigue than healthy individuals. In comparing CFS- and cancer-related fatigue, many similarities can be found. CFS comprises a complex of symptoms characterised by serious and debilitating, medically unexplained mental and physical fatigue of at least six months' duration, accompanied by a number of additional nonspecific symptoms including muscle pain, sleep disturbance, depression, and poor concentration [13]. No definitive treatment or aetiology has been established, and the available evidence suggests that CFS is heterogeneous and multicausal.

Fatigue has been documented as being difficult to define, and there is a lack of understanding of what it means to suffer from fatigue. There is also very little information regarding the meaning, impact, and experience of fatigue from the patient's perspective [14]. Some researchers have also found significant differences between patients and staff members in perception of symptom distress levels and occurrence [15]. To evaluate the problem in Sweden, a questionnaire was sent to 442 registered nurses with the aim of determining cancer nurses' views of the nature and causes of cancer-related fatigue and what, if any, nursing interventions they employed in the management of this problem. The response rate was 49%. The responses showed that these nurses regarded fatigue as the most common symptom in cancer patients but also that there were few established nursing interventions. In addition, the nurses desired further education and tools for evaluation of fatigue, its causes, and its treatment [16]. As health care providers we must be aware that fatigue may have a great impact on a patient's situation in physical, psychological, social, and existential dimensions.

The definition of fatigue

Cancer-related fatigue is a condition in which a person with cancer experiences an overwhelming and sustained sense of exhaustion and has a decreased capacity for physical and mental work. These situations of fatigue are not relieved by rest. "Normal fatigue" and fatigue associated with cancer or its treatment are not the same thing.

One problem when it comes to understanding cancer-related fatigue is perhaps that we have not yet reached a consensus about the definition of fatigue itself. There is also no clear and well-defined theoretical framework regarding the symptoms. Fatigue is an example of a complex phenomenon that is studied by many disciplines, e.g. nursing, psychology, and medicine, with no widely accepted definition [9]. Tiesinga et al. state that the number of definitions of a concept will increase as the number of disciplines investigating the problem increases. In the literature, definitions derived from the discipline of nursing are the most common (Table 1). The definitions of fatigue often allude to the multidimensional nature of the symptoms, and evidence for the occurrence of several different dimensions has been steadily accumulating over the past decade [17]. Nail and King's [18] definition implies that there is a voluntary component to fatigue: "Fatigue is a human response to the experience of having cancer and to undergoing treatment for cancer. Fatigue is a self-recognised phenomenon involving how the individual feels and how this feeling influences the activities in which one has chosen to engage." By this, they mean that an individual may feel fatigued and yet push himself to perform necessary activities. This is in contrast to weakness, which is a symptom produced by neurological syndromes in which there are no voluntary components in the performance of activities [19].

That fatigue is a multifactorial and multidimensional symptom complicates the situation. According to Winningham et al. [20] it is not known how fatigue is related to indicators of fatigue such as reduced energy expenditure, sleep disturbances, attention deficits, decreased endurance, somatic complaints (e.g. aching body, tired eyes), and weakness. Winningham et al. state that a major challenge in defining fatigue is differentiating among its causes, indicators, and effects.

Table 1. Examples of definitions of fatigue

Authors	Definition
Aistars [35] 1987	"Fatigue is a condition characterised by subjective feelings of generalised weariness, exhaustion, and lack of energy resulting from prolonged stress that is directly attributable to the disease process. The outcome is an impaired functional status which ultimately has an impact on quality of life."
Nail & King [18] 1987	"Fatigue is a human response to the experience of having cancer and to undergoing treatment for cancer. Fatigue is a self-recognised phenomenon involving how the individual feels and how this feeling influences the activities in which one has chosen to engage."
NANDA [53] 1993	"Fatigue is an overwhelming, sustained sense of exhaustion and decreased capacity for physical and mental work." *(NANDA=North American Nursing Diagnosis Association)*
Ream & Richardson [30] 1996	"Fatigue is a subjective, unpleasant symptom which incorporates total body feelings ranging from tiredness to exhaustion creating an unrelenting overall condition which interferes with individuals' ability to function to their normal capacity."
Piper [54] 1986	"Fatigue, from a nursing perspective, is identified as a subjective feeling of tiredness that is influenced by circadian rhythm. It can vary in unpleasantness, duration and intensity. When acute, it serves a protective function; when it becomes unusual, excessive or constant (chronic), it no longer serves this function and may lead to the aversion of activity with the desire to escape."
Piper, Lindsey & Dodd [32] 1987	"Fatigue is a subjective feeling of tiredness that is influenced by circadian rhythm; it can vary in unpleasantness, duration, and intensity. When acute, fatigue serves a protective function; when it is excessive or chronic, its function is unknown."

Fatigue can be used as a concept to describe a reduced capacity to sustain force or power output (physiological), a reduced capacity to perform multiple tasks over time (psychological), and simply a subjective experience of feeling exhausted, tired, weak or having a lack of energy [21].

The dimensions of fatigue

A dimension is a component of a complex concept [22]. Most definitions of fatigue allude to its multidimensionality and include a performance or work decrement dimension, a physical/physiological dimension, and a subjective or symptom/sensory dimension [23]. A concept analysis performed by Ream and Richardson suggested that fatigue is a holistic experience that permeates the entire body [24].

Many researchers stress the importance of the subjective dimension. Dimensions similar to those for pain have been suggested for fatigue, e.g. sensory, affective, behavioural, and physiological [23]. The definitions of fatigue and pain have several components in common, such as being subjective and being caused by several factors of both a physical and a psychological nature [8]. Pain is also defined as a subjective phenomenon by the International Association for Study in Pain (IASP): "Pain is an unpleasant sensory and emotional experience associated with actual or potential tissue damage, or described in terms of such damage" [25]. Glaus [5] has proposed that fatigue be defined based on an adaptation of McCaffrey's definition of pain [26]: "Fatigue is whatever the patient says it is, whenever the patient says it is." The dimensions of fatigue are not as well researched or as well conceptualised as the dimensions of pain, although similar dimensions have been proposed for both [23].

A few qualitative studies have been conducted with the purpose of exploring, in multiple dimensions, the experience of fatigue in cancer patients [6,7,27-30]. These studies indicate that fatigue is an experience of the whole person, i.e., body and mind, a complex phenomenon with physical, emotional, and mental sensations and a great impact on everyday functioning and perceived control. In one study the respondents described their fatigue as a process of 1) experiences (of loss, need, malaise, psychological stress, emotional affection, abnormal weakness, difficulties in taking initiative); 2) consequences (social limitations, affected self-esteem, affected quality of life); and 3) actions (coping). The respondents described their fatigue in more than one dimension, and the process contained a dynamic development within the categories: instead of expressing the experience of fatigue the respondents could express the consequences of fatigue or the actions related to these consequences [6]. This may indicate that it is not possible to isolate fatigue as only an experience. Because fatigue is a symptom that is hard to verbalise, it may be easier for the patient to explain the effects of the fatigue. Glaus et al. [7] conducted a study on 20 cancer patients and 20 healthy individuals using a grounded theory approach. They found that reports of fatigue/tiredness could be divided into expressions of physical, affective, and cognitive fatigue/tiredness. To structure this study, Glaus used the three steps that Bruera [31] used to explain pain: nociception, perception, and expression.

Fatigue is a complex phenomenon, and the separation of its causes and effects presents a chicken-and-egg dilemma. It may not always be easy to know whether fatigue is felt "in the body" or "in the mind". For example, if a person is feeling tired in the head (like a slight dizziness), should this be characterised as mental or physical fatigue? As it may be hard to know where the feeling is located (in the head or in the mind), it may be equally hard to know how it feels. There is little scientific insight into which dimensions should be classified as dimensions and which as subdimensions [9].

Theoretical foundations

Clarification of the meaning of fatigue is fundamental for the development of fatigue theories, and the strategies of developing a theory related to fatigue must be identified. The framework of Piper et al. [32], the Integrated Fatigue Model (IFM), is the most widely used theoretical framework of fatigue in cancer patients, and it is used to guide the selection of variables for study and the structure of the collection instruments [33]. This framework takes a deductive approach derived from the five disciplines that have investigated fatigue: psychology, physiology, ergonomics, medicine, and nursing. Piper et al. address many potential causes of fatigue and point out the importance of considering multiple aspects of the manifestation of fatigue. Because changes in biological and psychosocial patterns may influence the signs and symptoms of fatigue, it is important for health care providers to assess whether changes in preexisting patterns have occurred as a result of the illness or the treatment [34]. Using this framework health care providers can assess the possible causes of fatigue in specific patient situations and select appropriate interventions. Winningham et al. [20] state that one strength of the IFM is its usefulness to researchers in guiding the assessment of potential aetiological factors related to fatigue. The IFM also identifies factors that may influence the perceptions of fatigue in patients with cancer (see Fig. 1). Examples of other cancer-oriented frameworks are the Aistars Organizing Framework [35], Winningham's Psychobiologic-Entropy Hypothesis [20], and Cimprich's attentional theory [36-38].

The words used to describe fatigue

Because cancer-related fatigue is not like the normal fatigue that we all experience sometimes, there is a lack of nuance in the language used to describe the experience. The words that we are accustomed to using suddenly become insufficient. The descriptions may come from different dimensions of fatigue. This may mean that what the patient says can be interpreted as something other than fatigue. For example, it is easier for the caregiver to diagnose fatigue if a patient says he or she does not have any energy or feels weak than if the patient says he or she is listless or finds it difficult to think clearly. This implies that health care providers must listen very carefully to the patient's own descriptions of fatigue.
Cancer-related fatigue has been described by patients as tiredness, weakness, lack of energy, exhaustion, lethargy, depression, inability to concentrate, malaise, asthenia, boredom, sleepiness, lack of motivation, and decreased men-

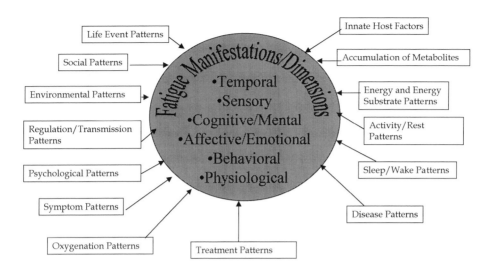

Fig. 1. Piper's integrated fatigue model. © 1997 Reproduced with permission, Barbara F. Piper, D.N.Sc, RN, AOCN, FAAN

tal status [20]. In the study of Magnusson et al. [6] the respondents tried to explain the experience of fatigue in one word, but not everyone could find a word for it. The words used were, for example, "listless", "sluggish", "faint", "despondent", "apathetic", "tired", "slack", "indifferent", and "paralysing fatigue". In the study of Hillfinger Messias et al. [28] the participants used words such as "beaten", "wiped out", "pooped", "real blah", "lousy", "drained", "sluggish", and "slumpish" as descriptions of fatigue.

Some studies have shown that patients often use metaphors instead of the term "fatigue" itself, for example, "my feet feel like lead" or "I couldn't run, my legs felt like spaghetti" [6]. From the same study there are statements from patients who are experiencing fatigue that we can use as examples to show how difficult it may be to recognise fatigue when it is explained from its different dimensions. For example, "You feel like a block of concrete", "I can't get started doing anything", "When I am walking I have to stop much more often, my feet start aching very soon", "I feel I forget a lot of things", "You feel as if you are inside a glass jar" and "I easily stagger and fall". There are a lot of differences in these statements, but it is possible to put all of them under the umbrella term "fatigue".

Diagnostic criteria

Although fatigue is recognised as a significant clinical problem, progress towards treatment has been hampered by a lack of consensus about definition and formal diagnosis [39]. We must also continuously encourage the patient to inform us if any adverse effects, including fatigue, have occurred. The more we show that we are interested in finding out how the patient is feeling from the start, the more we will get to know.

Cella et al. [39] present a draft list of diagnostic criteria that are intended to be inclusive of the various causes of fatigue (see Table 1 of the chapter by Cella et al. in this volume). They have also developed an interview guide to help ensure that the diagnosis of cancer-related fatigue is made correctly. It is of course important, as in all diagnostic procedures, that a standardised template be used to ensure that the patient's experience is interpreted correctly. However, one must also leave room for the sovereignty of the individual patient and his/her special story. Cella et al.'s "Diagnostic Interview Guide for Cancer-Related Fatigue" (CRF) (Draft 1998) comprises twelve questions aimed at the patient; at two points (after question 1 and 11) room is allowed to determine whether the response could be correlated with CRF or not. If not, the interview is interrupted, and another explanatory model must be found. The interview guide concludes with two questions that give the interviewer the opportunity to evaluate the estimate; in other words, if the patient can be given the diagnosis CRF or not.

A detailed characterisation of fatigue, coupled with an understanding of the most likely aetiological factors, is necessary to develop a therapeutic strategy. According to Portenoy and Itri a comprehensive assessment includes a description of fatigue-related phenomena, a physical examination, and a review of laboratory and imaging studies. These data may suggest plausible hypotheses concerning pathogenesis, which in turn may suggest appropriate strategies (see chapter by Portenoy and Itri in this volume).

Other characteristics are similarly important, for example, onset, duration, severity, daily pattern, time course, exacerbating and reducing factors, and distress associated with fatigue and the distinction between acute (of recent onset and anticipated to end in the near future) and chronic (weeks to months or longer) fatigue [40; chapter by Portenoy and Itri in this volume]. In 1988 Piper [41] undertook a review of the literature regarding the distinguishing characteristics of acute and chronic fatigue and summarised it in a table (Table 2). This table is still up to date and is very helpful as a clear demonstration of the differences.

Patient evaluation

For patients fatigue may be one of the most taxing and worrying symptoms, whereas we as health care providers sometimes underestimate the impact of the experience. This implies that fatigue may be ignored, with the result that patients may feel that they have not been given adequate care or have even been rejected. If interventions are to be implemented, measures must be available to study the effects of the interventions [42].

Table 2. Acute and chronic fatigue: Distinguishing characteristics (Piper 1988)

Characteristics	Acute Fatigue	Chronic fatigue
Purpose/Function	Protective	Unknown, may no longer be protective May be nonfunctional
Population at risk	Primarily healthy	Primarily clinical populations
Aetiology	Usually identifiable Usually involves a single mechanism or cause Often experienced in relation to some form of activity or exertion	May not be identifiable Usually multiple and additive causes Often experienced with no relation to activity or exertion
Perception	Normal, usual Expected/anticipated with respect to specific activities or forms Primarily localised to a specific body part or system Pleasant or unpleasant	Abnormal, unusual Excessive or disproportionate to past experience Generalised, whole body- mind sensation Unpleasant
Time dimension Onset	Rapid	Insidious, gradual Cumulative Threshold model
Duration	Short; days or weeks	Long; persists over time More than 1 month
Relief dimension	Usually alleviated by a good night's sleep, adequate rest, proper diet, exercise programme, or stress management techniques Resolves quickly	Not completely dispelled by these methods Does not resolve quickly
Impact on activities of daily living and quality of life	Minor, minimal	Major

Reproduced with permission from Piper B. Fatigue in cancer patients: Current perspectives on measurement and management [41].

Again, it is important to remember that fatigue is a subjective experience but must be measured by objective parameters. Normally, subjective fatigue correlates fairly well with its objective relative, e.g. when we are objectively tired, we often feel tired, too. However, there is no absolute relation between these two aspects, especially when we are talking about cancer-related fatigue or in some pathological cases. Patients with CFS describe feelings of muscle weariness or tiredness unrelated to objective measures of muscle fatigue. Wessley [43] and DeLuca et al. [44] found in their studies that CFS patients did not differ from control subjects on tasks of higher-order cognitive functioning, e.g. memory, even though they showed a high degree of subjective complaints of cognitive impairment. On the other hand, a depressed patient may not be able to embark on any physical or mental activity because the feelings of fatigue are so overwhelming. In a review Stone et al. [45] explain the subjective state as being characterised by a feeling of weariness, a perception of decreased capacity for physical or mental work, and an objective decrement in physical or mental performance with repeated or prolonged activity.

It is important to give the patient a chance to tell the health care provider if he or she is suffering from fatigue and, if so, how severe it is. The most frequently used method is to interview the patient about his or her situation and any changes that may have occurred since the last interview. The interviewer should ask the patient, and perhaps his or her significant others, questions about changes in the mood of the patient and his or her general situation or habits. The interviewer should also observe whether the patient looks tired and pale or whether he or she is slow in movements.

To encourage the patient to report fatigue, the health care provider should inform the patient about the symptoms of fatigue at the beginning of the disease or treatment period and monitor the situation continually from that point.

The health care provider needs to include all subjective and objective data that may influence the experience of fatigue for a patient. According to Piper [34] the subjective data should include an assessment of the fatigue's

- location;
- pattern;
- intensity;
- onset;
- duration;
- aggravating factors;
- associated symptoms;
- changes in usual pattern,

and the objective data should include

- a physical examination;
- a review of laboratory data;
- a review of medical and drug histories;
- assessment of environmental factors ;
- documentation of any changes in the patient's physical appearance, performance status, and ways of moving, talking, or interacting.

The experience of fatigue cannot be directly measured by an observer; it can only be assessed by self-report [45]. In this way, it is personally assessed by the individual patient. Therefore, it is necessary to characterise fatigue in the patient's own words [20]. The most commonly used instrument in the research literature is therefore a so-called "self-report instrument". But, technically, it is also possible to assess fatigue by interview or observation.

Recommendations for assessing fatigue vary according to the purpose of the assessment, and there is a great difference between the assessment of fatigue in clinical practice and in research. In clinical practice the focus is on efficiently obtaining information that is needed for patient care. It must also be simple to evaluate a symptom in practice. Validated multidimensional instruments provide a more sophisticated way of assessing fatigue, but they are hard to use in clinical practice because of time limitations and the burden on the patient.

Assessment strategies similar to those used for pain are also appropriate for fatigue [20]. One way is to ask the patient, "On a scale of 1 to 10, how much fatigue are you experiencing now?"

Portenoy and Itri suggest the routine use of three questions to help assess the severity of fatigue and its impact over time:
- Are you experiencing any fatigue?
- If so, how severe has it been, on average, during the past week, using a 0 to 10 scale?
- How does the fatigue interfere with your ability to function?

A detailed characterisation of fatigue, coupled with an understanding of the most likely aetiological factors, is necessary to develop a therapeutic strategy [40; chapter by Portenoy and Itri in this volume].

Winningham et al. [20] also state that, in addition to the level of fatigue, it is important to obtain information on the time pattern, the exacerbating and relieving factors, the impact of fatigue on day-to-day activities, the meaning of fatigue to the individual, and the cultural influences on expression of feelings of fatigue.

As an initial approach to cancer-related fatigue, efforts should be made to correct potential aetiologies. Portenoy and Itri [40] have constructed an algorithm for evaluation and management of cancer-related fatigue (see chapter by Portenoy and Itri in this volume). This kind of model helps to guide the health care provider through the evaluation of the patient's fatigue. The algorithm is broken down into different easy-to-follow steps. Using this approach reduces the risk of missing something in the evaluation.

The use of a health diary is becoming more and more common in the setting of nursing practice. According to Richardson [46] nurses have incorporated the diary into the treatment plan as a means of helping patients document their symptoms and the factors which have precipitated them, often with the aim of modifying particular health behaviours. Examples of symptoms that are suited to this kind of data collection are pain, nausea and fatigue.

In the diary the patient can enter many factors that may serve as the foundation of an evaluation of his or her situation. Examples of this include:
- when the fatigue occurred (time);
- how the fatigue occurred (in what context);
- degree of fatigue;
- type of fatigue;

- pattern of fatigue;
- if any measures are taken;
- if any measures taken had any results.

Using the diary as a basis the patient can then, together with the caregiver and any close relatives, make a thorough analysis of the pattern of fatigue, any risk factors for its occurrence, and how the fatigue should be handled. At the next visit the evaluation should be repeated and any measures taken should be evaluated. Richardson [46] states that the use of a diary may also be a method of data collection for research.

Assessment tools

Researchers may be interested in the distinct separation of fatigue sensations and responses to fatigue, obtaining data from a variety of different instruments, and comparing a variety of approaches to measure fatigue [20].

Fatigue is considered to be a multidimensional construct, but this is not always reflected in the choice of measurement strategies [33]. Available instruments can basically be divided into so-called unidimensional and multidimensional instruments. The response formats of these instruments include yes/no, Likert-type scales, and visual analogue scales.

Piper and associates were the first to propose a multidimensional measurement model for fatigue manifestations [32]. This model was strongly influenced by what was known about pain manifestations at the time. Today many instruments exist, but they do not always measure the same thing. Comparisons are hindered by the fact that there has been little standardisation of fatigue measurement between studies [4].

Fatigue is often included as a subscale in several cancer-specific quality of life measures. Examples of these instruments are the European Organisation for Research and Treatment of Cancer questionnaire (EORTC QLQ-C30) [47] and the Rotterdam Symptom Checklist (RSCL) [48]. There are also specific instruments for cancer-related fatigue, for example, the Functional Assessment of Cancer Therapy (FACT) [49], the Piper Fatigue Scale (PFS) [50], the Multi Fatigue Inventory (MFI-20) [51-52], and the Fatigue Assessment Questionnaire (FAQ) [1]. These instruments are multidimensional scales, and they attempt to gauge both the quality of the symptom and its severity.

It is necessary to use instruments with reliability and validity in research if we wish to obtain credible and generalisable results. But we also need an instrument that can be used in daily practice. Perhaps some kind of global estimation of multidimensional fatigue will be a goal for the future.

All patients have an upper limit for the amount of fatigue they can tolerate without a change in their quality of life. This limit varies according to the goal of the treatment, the stage of the disease, the applicable social factors, and individual differences. It is important to respect each patient's individual limit. We want our patients to be in good general condition and to have a high quality of life while at the same time being able to carry out oncological treatment according to plan. This necessitates mutual discussion with emphasis on the individual patient's disease, treatment plan, and quality of life.

References

1   Glaus A. Fatigue in patients with cancer. Analysis and assessment. Berlin: Springer-Verlag, 1998
2   Barnish L Fatigue and the cancer patient. Br Nurs 1994; 3: 806-9
3   Grandjean E. Fatigue: its physiological and psychological significance. Ergonomics 1968; 11: 427-36
4   Lewis G, Wessley S. The epidemiology of fatigue: more questions than answers. J Epidemiol Community Health 1992; 46: 92-7
5   Glaus A. Assessment of fatigue in cancer and non-cancer patients and in healthy individuals. Support Care Cancer 1993; 1: 305-15
6   Magnusson K, Möller A, Ekamn T, Wallgren A. A qualitative study to explore the experience of fatigue in cancer patients. Eur Cancer Care 1999; 8: 224-32
7   Glaus A, Crow R, Hammond S. A qualitative study to explore the concept of fatigue/tiredness in cancer patients and in healthy individuals. Eur Cancer Care 1996; 5 (suppl 2): 8-23
8   Kaasa S, Loge J, Knobel H, et al. Fatigue. Measures and relation to pain. Acta Anaesthesiol Scand 1999; 43: 939-47
9   Tiesinga L, Dassen T, Halfens R. Fatigue: A summary of the definitions, dimensions and indicators. Nurs Diagn 1996; 7: 51-62
10 Milligan R, Pugh L. Fatigue during the childbearing period. In: Fitzpatrick JJ, Stevenson JS, eds. Annual Review of Nursing Research, Vol. 12. New York: Springer Verlag, 1994; 33-49
11 Freel M, Hart L. Study of fatigue phenomena of multiple sclerosis patients (USDHEW Grant No. 5R02-NU-00534-02). University of Iowa Division of Nursing, Iowa City, 1977
12 Krupp L, LaRocca N, Muir-Nash J, et al. The fatigue severity scale: Application to patients with multiple sclerosis and systematic lupus erythematosus. Arch Neurol 1989; 46: 1121-3
13 Holmes G, Kaplan J, Gantz N, et al. Chronic fatigue syndrome: a working case definition. Ann Intern Med 1988; 108: 387-9
14 Pearce S, Richardson A. Fatigue in cancer: a phenomenological perspective. Eur J Cancer Care 1996; 5: 111-5
15 Vogelzang N, Breitbart W, Cella D, et al. Patient, caregiver, and oncologist perceptions of cancer-related fatigue: results of a tripart assessment survey. Semin Hematol 1997; 34 (suppl 2): 4-12
16 Magnusson K, Karlsson E, Palmblad C, Leitner C, Paulson A. Swedish nurses' estimation of fatigue as a symptom in cancer patients - report on a questionnaire. Eur Cancer Care 1997; 6: 186-91
17 Richardson A, Ream E, Wilson-Barnett J. Fatigue in patients receiving chemotherapy: Patterns of change. Cancer Nurs 1998; 21; 17-30
18 Nail L, King K. Fatigue. Semin Oncol Nurs 1987; 3; 257-62
19 Gordon M. Differential diagnosis of weakness: a common geriatric symptom. Geriatrics 1986; 41: 75-9
20 Winningham M, Nail L, Barton Burke M, et al. Fatigue and the cancer experience: The state of the knowledge. Oncol Nurs Forum 1994; 21: 23-36
21 Wessely S. The epidemiology of chronic fatigue syndrome. Epidemiol Rev 1995; 17: 1-13
22 Polit D, Hungler B. Nursing research: Principles and methods (5th ed.). Philadelphia: Lippincott, 1995

23 Piper B. Measuring fatigue. In: Frank-Stromborg M, Olsen J, eds. Instruments for clinical health-care research. London: Jones and Barlett Publishers, 1997; 482-96.
24 Ream E, Richardson A. Fatigue: a concept analysis. Int J Nurs Stud 1996; 33: 519-29
25 International Association for the Study of Pain. Pain term: a list with definitions and notes on usage. Pain 1979; 6: 249-52
26 McCaffrey M. Nursing management of the patient with pain. Philadelphia: Lippincott, 1979
27 Ferrell B, Grant M, Dean G, Funk B, Ly J. "Bone Tired": The experience of fatigue and its impact on quality of life. Oncol Nurs Forum 1996; 23: 1539-47
28 Hillfinger Messias D, Yeager K, Dibble S, Dodd M. Patients' perspective of fatigue while undergoing chemotherapy. Oncol Nurs Forum 1997; 24: 43-8
29 Krishnasamy M. Exploring the nature and impact of fatigue in advanced cancer. Int J Palliat Nurs 1997; 3: 126-31
30 Ream E, Richardson A. Fatigue in patients with cancer and chronic obstructive airways disease: a phenomenological enquiry. Int Nurs Stud 1997; 34: 44-53
31 Bruera E. New developments in the assessment of pain in cancer patients. Support Care Cancer 1994; 2: 312-8
32 Piper B, Lindsey A, Dodd M. Fatigue mechanisms in cancer patients: Developing nursing theory. Oncol Nurs Forum 1987; 14: 17-23
33 Richardson A. Fatigue in cancer patients: a review of the literature. Eur Cancer Care 1995; 4: 20-32
34 Piper B. Fatigue: Current bases for practice. In: Funk S, Tournquist E, eds. Key aspects of comfort. Berlin, Heidelberg, New York: Springer Verlag, 1989; 187-99
35 Aistars J. Fatigue in the cancer patient: A conceptual approach to a clinical problem. Oncol Nurs Forum 1987; 14: 25-30
36 Cimprich B. Attentional fatigue following breast cancer surgery. Res Nurs Health 1992; 15: 199-207
37 Cimprich B. A theoretical perspective on attention and patient education. Adv Nursing Sci 1992; 14: 39-51
38 Cimprich B. Development of an intervention to restore attention in cancer patients. Cancer Nurs 1993; 16: 83-92
39 Cella D, Peterman A, Passik S, et al. Progress towards guidelines for the management of fatigue. Oncology, 1998; 12: 1-9
40 Porteny R, Itri L. Cancer-related fatigue: Guidelines for evaluation and management. Oncologist 1999; 4: 1-10
41 Piper B. Fatigue in cancer patients: Current perspectives on measurement and management. Fifth National Conference on Cancer Nursing. Monograph on nursing management of common problems: State of the art. New York: American Cancer Society, 1988; 24-36
42 Loge J, Kaasa S. Fatigue and cancer – prevalence, correlates and measurement. Progr Palliat Care, 1998; 6: 43-47
43 Wessely S. Chronic fatigue. In: Greenwood R et al, eds. Neurological rehabilitation. Edinburgh: Churchill Livingstone, 1993
44 DeLuca J, Johnson SK, Beldowicz D, Natelson BH. Neuropsychological impairments in chronic fatigue syndrome, multiple sclerosis, and depression. J Neurol Neurosurg Psychiatry 1995; 58: 38-42
45 Stone P, Richards M, Hardy J. Fatigue in patients with cancer. Eur J Cancer 1998; 34: 1670-6
46 Richardson A. The health diary: an example of its use as a data collection method. J Adv Nurs 1994; 19: 782-91
47 Aaronson NK, Ahmedzai S, Bergman B, et al. The European Organisation for Research and Treatment of Cancer QLQ-C30: a quality of life instrument for use in international clinical trials in oncology. J Natl Cancer Inst 1993; 85: 365-76

48 de Haes JCJM, van Kippenberg FCE, Neijt JP. Measuring psychological and physical distress in cancer patients: structure and application of the Rotterdam Symptom Checklist. Br J Cancer 1990; 62: 1034-8

49 Cella D, Tulsky D, Gray G, et al. The Functional Assessment of Cancer Therapy Scale: development and validation of the general measure. J Clin Oncol 1993; 11: 570-9

50 Piper B, Lindsey A, Dodd M, Ferketich S, Paul S, Weller S. The development of an instrument to measure the subjective dimension of fatigue. In: Funk S, Tournquist E, eds. Key aspects of comfort. Berlin, Heidelberg, New York: Springer Verlag, 1989; 199-216

51 Smets EMA, Garssen B, Bonke B, de Haes JCJM. The Multidimensional Fatigue Inventory (MFI). Psychometric qualities of an instrument to assess fatigue. J Psychosom Res 1995; 39: 315-25

52 Smets EMA, Garssen B, Cull A, de Haes JCJM. Application of the multidimensional fatigue inventory (MFI-20) in cancer patients receiving radiotherapy. Br J Cancer 1996; 73: 241-5

53 NANDA. Fatigue. In: McFarland G, McFarlane E, eds. Nursing diagnosis and intervention, 2nd ed. St. Louis: Mosby, 1993; 288-92

54 Piper B. Fatigue. In: Carrieri VK, Lindsey AM, West CW, eds. Pathophysiological phenomena in nursing: Human responses to illness. Philadelphia: WB Saunders, 1986; 219-34

ESO Scientific Updates, Vol. 5
Fatigue and Cancer
M. Marty and S. Pecorelli, editors
© 2001 Elsevier Science B.V. All rights reserved

Assessment of Fatigue in Cancer Patients

Andrew Bottomley

Quality of Life Unit, European Organisation for Research and Treatment of Cancer, Brussels, Belgium

Introduction

Fatigue is without doubt one of the more common symptoms experienced by cancer patients, presenting a challenging and complex phenomenon for measurement [1-4]. The effects of fatigue on patient quality of life are considerable, influencing most domains. For example, fatigue can influence the ability to socialise with family and friends and to continue a normal sexual relationship, it can impair cognitive processes and/or contribute to mood disorders [5-13].

Studies have shown that fatigue correlates directly with overall quality of life, greater fatigue often leading to poorer outcomes. A considerable number of studies reported in the literature in the last decade stress the complex problem faced by cancer patients experiencing fatigue either when undergoing treatments and/or following a course of treatment [12,14,15]. Further, fatigue can continue for many years once treatment has ceased [16], and in patients with progressive disease fatigue can simply lead to a loss of overall quality of life that is limiting in the extreme. However, there is still a great deal to understand about the effects of fatigue on cancer patients. While researchers continue to develop new treatments and approaches that may have benefits in terms of survival, it is important that health workers continue to understand how fatigue affects cancer patient quality of life.

Over the past decade researchers and clinicians have become increasingly aware of the negative influence of fatigue on quality of life, devoting considerable time to the development of tools to assess fatigue. Some authors, such as Simon and Zittoun [17], suggest that this increased interest in fatigue and its effect on cancer patients is due to other troublesome symptoms such as nausea and pain, claiming that when these are controlled, patients naturally focus on other problems.

However, whatever the reason for the increased interest, researchers are still asking basic questions such as, How is fatigue assessed? Why isn't there a

Address for correspondence: A. Bottomley, EORTC Data Center, Avenue E. Mounier 83, 1200 Brussels, Belgium. Tel.: +32-2-7741661, fax: +32-2-7794568, e-mail: abo@eortc.be

gold standard to measure or compare fatigue? What are the key dimensions of fatigue? For example, should researchers focus on the physical, the spiritual, the emotional or all of these possible dimensions at the same time? Perhaps researchers should keep the assessment of fatigue simple and brief by focusing on a single question such as "Do you feel tired?" If researchers and clinicians do choose measures to examine fatigue, are there different measures which should be used with different cancer patients and at different times in the disease cycle? Even if information is collected from patients about fatigue, how would researchers interpret this? For example, what level of score on any given fatigue measure would suggest clinical intervention? What are the key properties in a fatigue measurement that researchers should look for?

Clearly, these are key questions many researchers and clinicians face when working with patients who may suffer from fatigue. If a significant, robust and reliable conclusion about the fatigue experienced is to be made, it is essential that robust measures to assess patient fatigue and to make meaningful judgements are available. This chapter therefore aims to provide a brief overview of important issues in the development of fatigue-measuring tools, and will highlight some of the currently used measures. Hopefully this will provide some insight into the possibility of using certain fatigue measurements in clinical and research practice.

Some key methodological issues in measures used to assess fatigue

There are a number of important reasons why fatigue should be assessed. When the problem of fatigue is examined at the research level, fatigue assessments should be part of the more global quality of life assessment because these two factors are interrelated. As is noted in the literature of the last decade, much can be learned from evaluating new and developing treatments for patient fatigue in relation to overall quality of life. This is particularly true in clinical trials as, increasingly, more toxic drugs and challenging interventions are given to patients in the hope of a greater improvement in survival or other end points. This is supported by an increasing body of evidence that suggests fatigue to be a key concern of patients [18]. Frequently any medical interventions are considered in terms of positive and negative results due to their impact on patient fatigue [19,20].

With inpatients undergoing treatment in palliative care trials, issues such as fatigue management become a hugely important matter. Interventions to reduce or improve the impact on fatigue can be a key outcome for these patients [21].

There is increasing evidence that greater knowledge of patient fatigue can be useful in designing new approaches and interventions, giving patients the skills to help reduce fatigue [22]. For example, Smets et al. [23] observed in a sample of 250 cancer patients that fatigue during radiotherapy increased as treatment progressed but decreased after the treatment ended, suggesting that preparatory information to help new patients cope could be useful prior to treatment commencement. New interventions are being examined that aim to provide patients with more effective skills to cope with fatigue. For example, Dimeo et al. [24] examined levels of fatigue in 59 patients undergoing high-dose chemotherapy randomised to receive either a 30-minute daily exercise session on a bike or no intervention. Using the Profile of Mood States (POMS) tool, they conclude that exercise reduces levels of fatigue and could help patients cope with the distress of the treatment The researchers have begun large-scale randomised trials to provide stronger evidence for their position.

A number of psychological interventions suggest some coping-skills training approaches could be useful in helping patients cope with fatigue [25,26]. Bjordal [27] found in a study of long-term patients with head and neck cancer that those patients who underwent hyperfractionated radiotherapy enjoyed a better quality of life and less fatigue than patients who underwent conventional radiotherapy. This leads to a consideration of social support and other interventions to help the conventional radiotherapy group cope with greater fatigue and poorer quality of life. Many of the results obtained help to increase the understanding of fatigue, relying heavily on the use of measures to provide insight into these new interventions.

When considered at the individual patient level, it is important that a patient's level of fatigue can be assessed by a single clinician. This knowledge is essential for the overall care of the patient [28], helping the clinician in selecting appropriate interventions that may reduce fatigue and lead to an overall improvement in the patient's quality of life. Clinicians have a substantial impact in not just treating but in guiding patients. There is evidence that cancer patients do initiate their own self-coping mechanisms such as nutritional interventions and symptom relief strategies to deal with fatigue. However, these mechanisms are largely ineffective. For example, patients are often seen choosing poor nutritional approaches in the incorrect belief that these will help, and adopting strategies which in fact can aggravate fatigue symptoms rather than reduce them [29].

It is also a possibility that assessing fatigue can increase the level of interaction and communication between clinician and patient, leading to more collaborative treatment and care. Evidence from quality of life assessments in cancer patients demonstrates that patients are more satisfied when clinicians inquire about quality of life issues. Further, there is greater satisfaction in the consultation process for clinician and patient if interactions are recorded, along with evidence of greater awareness on the part of the clinician in the quality of life issues facing the patient [30].

What are the key properties of fatigue measures?

A considerable number of measures have been developed to assess fatigue [31-34]. However, like pain, fatigue is a complex, subjective phenomenon that can only be measured by self-report assessment. Researchers have long agreed that patients are the best judges of their own condition. However, a debate over the need to develop a test for fatigue has been ongoing for considerable time. In fact, Richardson [1] points out that in 1921 Musci wrote an article in the *British Journal of Psychology* entitled "Is a fatigue test possible?" In that article he states that "the term [fatigue] be absolutely banished from scientific discussion, and consequently that attempts to measure fatigue be abandoned". Many researchers still argue that better assessment tools than those available at present are urgently needed and significant methodological rigour must accompany the development of these new tools to produce meaningful and valid results.

Reliability and validity

An important issue in any measuring instrument development is the need to ensure that the measure fulfils the basic psychometric criteria of reliability and validity. In brief, reliability refers to the tool's ability to constantly expose the issue in question, producing reproducible and consistent results. There are various ways to assess reliability; one of the most common is the test-retest, whereby the patient, with a given level of fatigue, is assessed and then reassessed a few days later. All things being considered, and as long as there are no major interventions such as new treatments, it would be generally expected that similar scores would be demonstrated on both assessments, suggesting a reliable level of agreement. Other forms of reliability have also been used, such as inter-rater and equivalent forms, and the reader is referred to other texts for a detailed analysis [35].

In the case of validity, the essence is focused on ensuring that the measure does indeed detect what it is designed to detect. In referring to validity, it is important to note that there are several types of validity, all of which can have important implications for a measure used. For example, a measure must have content validity. This is a critical aspect related to the tool's validity to measure the patient population problem/difficulty. One would expect that there is appropriate coverage of items and that these are specific to the issue of concern, in this case fatigue. Face validity is also important and a related concept. In essence it asks about the measure's validity in terms of the appearance. Experts reviewing the measures and describing the validity of the measure often report on this. An effective measure of validity is criterion – a method of comparing the measure against another known value or believed true score.

However, with a fatigue measure this is difficult, as no gold standard allowing direct comparison exists. Because other fatigue measures are available it is possible to make some comparisons between measuring tools, collecting empirical evidence to support the notion that a certain measure has meaning. Finally, construct validity is essential for any measure. This involves the development of a theoretical framework for the issue, and generally examines the concepts using correlation analysis to further refine the model. Many methods are used to provide construct analysis, such as known group comparisons, convergent validity and discriminate validity. Readers are referred to several text books on these topics including the work by Fayers and Machin [35].

Cultural relevance

One essential element in using a tool to assess fatigue, particularly in the European setting, is the consideration of tool validity in terms of culture. All too frequently measures are developed in a single language (culture) and then, if need be, translated into a target language with little consideration for cultural factors that influence everyday life, the way events are interpreted and how meaning is determined [36]. Culture has a substantial effect on everybody, yet to many the effect is unrecognised. When developing a new measure of fatigue in a country, for example the USA, it could be possible that the political, social and cultural pressures cause researchers and patients to empathise a certain aspect of fatigue as more important than may be seen in other countries. There is considerable evidence to suggest, for example, that measures developed in the USA need revision and adaptation for use in a European setting [37,38].

Further, it may be that in any particular culture the physical aspects of fatigue are seen as more important than in another culture that views the social or psychological aspects of fatigue as more important. This could lead to the development of a tool that would focus on these issues with less cross-cultural significance. In fact, not only could dimensions of fatigue be different, but it is possible that the weight individuals put to dimensions of fatigue could also be different. For example, some cultures may accept that fatigue is a normal consequence of cancer and its treatment, while other cultures may reject this notion. There is considerable evidence from quality of life research over the past decade confirming the significant variations in how aspects of quality of life – social, psychological and physical – are considered in different countries and cultures. Therefore, it is reasonable to assume that fatigue is also influenced by cultural factors. Clearly this aspect would benefit from more extensive research.

Fortunately, quality of life researchers have long recognised the problem of cultural variance, developing ways to ensure appropriateness of assessment tools. At the simplest level, measures are translated and hopefully pilot-tested to ensure the adequacy of the translation. While this has limited impact on establishing cultural validity, it at least ensures the tool is translated appropriately and is acceptable to patients. An optimal and more detailed approach is to develop the measure at the same time in not just a single country but in different countries, ensuring that there is validity of measurement across cultures. However, this methodology is vastly expensive, time-consuming and a significant administrative task, but one which creates robust measures such as the EORTC QLQ-30 and WHO measures. If measuring tools are to make meaningful conclusions in fatigue assessment or advocate interventions, cultural validity must be ensured.

Acceptability

One issue of key concern in the assessment of fatigue is making sure any tool developed is focused and, ideally, is easy for the patient to complete. Brevity is preferred where cancer patients are experiencing fatigue. While it is acknowledged that there is a loss of sensitivity in shorter scales and measures, researchers have ensured, with briefer scales, that key data is actually collected without overburdening the patient. The following review highlights to what extent selected fatigue measures have addressed the issues outlined above.

Measures of fatigue

The Rhoten Fatigue Scale [39]

The Rhoten Fatigue Scale is a single-item fatigue tool. The most important advantage of single-item measurement is that patients experience very little burden in terms of completion effort. Rhoten produced a measure that assesses subjective fatigue on a ten-point scale from *not tired* to *total exhaustion*. However, the problem with this measure lies in its development, where general postsurgical patients were used. Although there is some limited evidence of validity of the Rhoten Scale in cancer patients [40], the type of fatigue may differ in a cancer patient population. Further, one general limitation of any single-item measuring tool is the unidimensionality of the tool. In this case, it is possible that the Rhoten measure picks up not only fatigue but also elements of depression [40], a condition frequently associated with fatigue [12].

As the single-item Rhoten Scale cannot be evaluated against other forms for statistical reliability, the results may be problematic. For example, a critical argument for the validity of multi-item scales is the use of inter-item correlation tests. Because these cannot be undertaken on the Rhoten or any other single-item scale, they represent a major limitation. Given that patient populations may have different opinions on the actual questions asked, there is also a large number of random variations in a single-item measure. In multi-item measures higher reliability can be achieved. In addition, greater precision may be seen in multi-item measures than on a single scale, like the Rhoten Scale, where levels of fatigue are better discriminated. Some authors, such as Jacobsen and Stein [41], argue that due to the format a single-item measure only provides the most perfunctory information about patients' experience with fatigue.

The Piper Fatigue Self-Report Scale [42]

The Piper Fatigue Self-Report Scale was originally a two-form measure: one 42-item tool measured multidimensional aspects of fatigue – temporal, sensory, effective – on visual analogue scales designed to measure usual patterns of fatigue against any changes experienced six months prior to diagnosis or treatment. In addition, a 40-item scale, using essentially the same items, aimed to measure the present level of fatigue rather than past levels. The measure, developed using cancer patients, has been confirmed in review literature by an expert fatigue panel as valid, with good correlation with other measures, for example, the Profile of Mood States (POMS) [43].

However, while this measure has been used in studies with cancer patients [44], some authors argue that the measure can be too much of a burden for these patients [5]. In addition, several authors suggest that the items on the scale may be confounded by patient reaction to symptoms and their impact on daily living rather than assessing fatigue *per se*. It should also be noted that a number of patients find this scale difficult to complete, partly due to its complicated format [41,45]. An important point is that the wording of items and the response choice presumes that all patients are currently experiencing fatigue. Therefore, the tool can only be used to reliably measure patients who are first screened.

Piper et al. [31] undertook further developmental work to shorten the scale. A mail survey of 2250 US breast cancer survivors was conducted. Of the 32% (715) who responded only 382 were suitable for psychometric analysis. Factor analysis indicated that nearly half of the items on the measure could be dropped, leaving 22 items focusing on behavioural, affective, sensory and cognitive subscales. However, an important limitation of the assessment of the new Piper scale is that, while the sample size was adequate for factor analysis, the patient population was very self-selected – mainly US, affluent breast cancer survivors. It is likely that the dimensions of fatigue and scores obtained for these patients are different from other patients. Because this is significantly important to other cultures, it is likely that more testing of the measure will be undertaken to ascertain its validity in cross-cultural populations.

The Pearson-Byars Fatigue Checklist [46]

The Pearson-Byars Fatigue Checklist, developed to assess fatigue in healthy military personnel, is a brief 13-item measure with reliable internal consistency (alpha = 0.82-0.92). Used in a number of early cancer studies, the checklist proved to have the ability to discriminate between healthy volunteers and patients. The main concern centres on the measure's development in a vastly different population to cancer patients, and the issue of fatigue, as discussed, may have little bearing on the fatigue issues experienced by cancer patients; for example, malaise is not covered by the tool. The wording of the items, developed in the 1950s by US researchers, would be unsuitable for a European population today: for example, *fairly well*, *pooped*, *quite fresh*. It is reasonable to say that some of the words are perhaps less used in today's society, or have variant cultural meanings. The available literature suggests further, extensive development of this tool before use in a European setting.

The Multidimensional Fatigue Inventory [47]

The Multidimensional Fatigue Inventory (MFI) measure, specifically designed for use in cancer patients, covers five dimensions of fatigue: general, physical, reduced activity, reduced motivation and mental fatigue. Each of the 20 items is presented on a five-point scale where the patient is required to answer to what extent a particular question applies. The form can usually be completed in 10 minutes or less. The measure has demonstrated good internal consistency (alpha = 0.8) with construct validity, assessed during the initial validation study using cancer patients, groups of students, training clinicians, chronic fatigue patients and army recruits [47].

The 111 cancer patients were a heterogeneous sample of Dutch nationals attending outpatient radiotherapy at the time of assessment. In testing construct validity the cancer patients reported more fatigue than the non-cancer groups, although surprisingly this difference was minimal in the student population in the general fatigue subscale. Smets [47] suggests this may be attributed to the fact that the students have an active social life and thus have high levels of general fatigue. In addition, convergent validity was seen when comparing the MFI with a visual analogue scale, a measure that simply asks subjects to rate their levels of fatigue in the past week. Additional work on divergent validity has yet to be completed. No examination of test-retest is reported to support evidence of reliability.

The Fatigue Symptom Inventory [34]

The Fatigue Symptom Inventory, developed in the US specifically for cancer patients, is a brief 13-item measure aimed to examine both the intensity and duration of fatigue. The measure was initially developed by reviewing the literature and selecting relevant items. These were then given to cancer health care workers, 15 cancer patients and some non-cancer patients for review. From this, a number of revisions were made to the preliminary measure. Hann et al. [34] do not give an explicit explanation as to the nature, extent or reasons for the changes. However, the inventory seems a reasonable tool to develop face validity. The validation part of the study focused only on patients with breast cancer: those who were on treatment (n=117), those who had completed treatment (n=113), and a control group with no history of cancer (n=94).

The measure demonstrates good evidence of validity on convergent correlation with established measures of fatigue including POMS-F and the SF 36 vitality scale, and sensitivity. The scale can also discriminate between healthy volunteers and cancer patients. However, poor estimates of test-retest scores indicate that the measure may not reliably measure fatigue across either short (2-4 weeks) or longer periods of time (4-6 weeks). This renders the scale unsuitable for measuring fatigue in a repeated fashion, such as monitoring changes in fatigue over courses of cancer therapy or in the clinical research setting when trying to evaluate the effects of one treatment/intervention against another.

Also important is the limitation that the measure was developed for mainly female Caucasian breast cancer patients; this would suggest more validation work is required before use in other population groups and cultures such as are seen in the European setting. Another important factor in any measurement of fatigue is the acceptability of the tool to cancer patients. It is reported that to ensure a large enough sample of patients who have completed treatment an additional centre be involved. Initially, 29% of patients refused to participate. A detailed reason is not provided. While in general it appears that compliance was not an overall significant problem, there may need to be future work on the acceptability of the measure to different patient groups, such as those patients taken off treatment.

The Brief Fatigue Inventory [48]

The Brief Fatigue Inventory is a recent US addition to fatigue-measuring tools, based on the view that few measures in use are valid for cancer patients and many of those have limitations [48]. The scale was preliminarily developed on a mixed population. The initial stages included collection of data on fatigue using information from the *Wisconsin Fatigue Study*, in which 249 patients and healthy subjects were interviewed by means of an *ad hoc* measure. This provided tentative data on important aspects of fatigue. However, the sample had a considerable mix of patients including those with psychiatric disorders (29%). Only 27% of the sample were cancer patients. The authors concluded, on the basis of this work, that a more formal literature review was required for development of the Brief Fatigue Inventory.

The Brief Fatigue Inventory was subsequently developed from a review of the literature. It comprises nine items measured on a 10-point scale. Three items ask the patient to measure the severity of the fatigue and six items ask about the degree of fatigue the patient has experienced in the last 24 hours. The final validation study was conducted with 290 healthy US volunteers and 305 cancer patients, mainly haematological cancer patients (lymphoma and leukaemia) as well as patients with breast, gastrointestinal, genitourinary and gynaecological cancers, receiving either inpatient or outpatient treatment.

The results suggest the measure is highly acceptable to patients, with only five patients refusing to complete the tool. The measure demonstrates significant levels of validity, with good correlation with the POMS-F ($r=0.84$) subscale and the FACT-F ($r=0.88$) subscale. Evidence of discriminate validity was noted with significant correlation with the Brief Fatigue Inventory and haemoglobin levels ($r=-0.36$).

However, it must be considered that this measure was developed using a US sample, and at present is only available in a single language. Some cultural validation in other settings is needed. There may also be the problem of such a short time frame (i.e., 24-hour assessment of fatigue); this may fail to detect the true effects of the treatment and levels of fatigue, and pick up unstable variability from day to day.

The Schwartz Cancer Fatigue Scale [5]

The Schwartz Cancer Fatigue Scale, a recent arrival from the US, is a measure consisting of 28 items specific to the cancer patient, scored on a five-point Likert scale. The development of the tool followed an extensive literature search and item generation. Both patients and health care professionals were used to establish content validity before a population of mixed cancer patients, off treatment and undergoing treatment, was used to collect psychometric data. Initial factor analysis suggested that the tool has four distinct fatigue factors: physical, emotional, cognitive and temporal. The internal consistency was reported to be as high as 0.96. However, the scale development was limited in that no test-retest was performed, making it difficult to establish whether the instrument is responsive to change. Further, it is not clear if the tool can discriminate between different populations; this questions the construct validity. There was no other measure used with the tool to provide evidence of criterion validity. It is not clear how patients accepted the tool, or if patients found it took excessive time to complete, or if there is a degree of missing data. The measure was developed only in American English for a US population.

Quality of life measures with specific fatigue scales

Profile of Mood States - Fatigue and Vigour subscales [43]

The Profile of Mood States, extensively used in the US in many research studies with cancer patients [19,20,49], is a 65-item general measuring tool with significant reliability and validity. The measure has two subscales that may assess fatigue: *POMS Fatigue* and *Vigour*. The fatigue subscale consists of seven, and the vigour subscale of eight items. The wording of the items represents a challenge to the translator. For example, the scales use idiomatic words such as *full of pep*, *sluggish*, and *bushed*.

However, POMS has been used in many studies researching cancer patient quality of life, and in fatigue studies [12]. Significant data from the US studies is available for comparison with various cancer population groups: chemotherapy, radiotherapy and palliative care. However, some authors point out that there may be some problems with the fatigue subscale, given that the pattern of relationship between this scale, the vigour subscale and other measures of mood, symptoms and functional status is not consistent [1]. Importantly, it could be argued that the fatigue subscale detects symptoms of cancer as opposed to fatigue itself, given that several items on this scale are considered physical in nature. Further, some authors argue that the POMS is too great a burden for patients, particularly those suffering from fatigue [50,51].

The SF 36 - Fatigue subscale [52]

The Short Form 36 is a self-report measure containing eight individual sub-scales representing general areas of health status: emotional, physical and social well-being. The scale, initially developed on a US population of non-cancer patients derived from the medical outcomes study programme on research, including work on the nature and intensity of fatigue, has been extensively elaborated and tested and frequently used in US clinical trials. The SF 36 has an additional energy/fatigue subscale which consists of four items assessing how much time the individual has felt or experienced fatigue during a previous four-week period. These items ask respondents, among other things, if they felt *full of pep, had a lot of energy, felt tired*, or *felt worn out*. The fatigue subscale has been shown to discriminate between cancer patients and non-cancer patients [53]. However, while the measure has been used in some cancer trials to assess fatigue [54], it is not often used to assess cancer patients. Rather, it is a generic instrument more than a cancer-specific tool; thus it can lack the necessary sensitivity to detect certain treatment differences and is unsuitable for use in older patients [55]. Some researchers and clinicians have avoided using the measure with cancer patients because of some evidence of problems with the *physical functioning* scale [35], as well as challenges in translation [37,38] and sensitivity to variability using different modes of administration [56].

The EORTC QLQ-C30

The EORTC QLQ-C30, an integrated system for assessing quality of life in cancer patients, incorporates a brief fatigue scale among its multidimensional measurements designed for use in a wide range of cancer patients. To date over 1800 studies have used the EORTC QLQ-30. The measure, developed initially in 1987 as a 36-item tool, was later refined into a three-item third version in 1993. The early versions of the tool included a review of the literature and development and testing in a cross-cultural sample of lung cancer patients in 13 countries. This established face and content validity with cancer patients and health care professionals. The psychometric validation study indicated that the measure was acceptable across cultures. A significant level of reliability was seen with the fatigue subscale, with coefficients of alpha 0.80 and above. Patient acceptability of the tool is high, with less than 2% of missing data from the entire measure.

The fatigue subscale is a brief measure with three items, asking, *have you felt weak, did you need a rest* and *have you felt tired*. These items are based on the perception that fatigue is caused by the disease process. It appears that these items focus on the physical aspect of fatigue. The fatigue subscale has proved that it is able to discriminate between healthy patients and those with cancer [57] and between those with advanced versus non-advanced cancer. Evidence also exists for the ability of the subscale to discriminate between various cancer diseases. In addition, a clinical trial conducted by Glimelius et al.

[58] found that the QLQ-C30 could discriminate between patients whose hae-moglobin levels improved following treatment with epoetin and those with no haemoglobin improvement. In fact, it appears that an increase in haemoglobin levels is related to an improvement in quality of life and fatigue.

The EORTC QLQ-C30 is available in 38 languages. Given its wide accep-tance it represents a useful tool to specifically assess fatigue in cancer patients [59,60] with considerable literature reporting on fatigue problems of cancer and its treatment [61-63]. The strength of the EORTC QLQ-C30 measure rests in its development in the context of establishing cross-cultural validity, good inter-nal consistency and brevity. However, while the fatigue subscale is robust, the QLQ-C30 was designed for use in groups rather than individual patients. While the internal consistency is high, it is not as high as one would ideally require for the assessment of fatigue at the level of the individual patient. While the scale measures the intensity of fatigue, Hann et al. [34] noted that it does not measure fatigue duration and the EORTC believe there is a need for a more robust measure of fatigue and are currently developing one.

The FACT - Fatigue and Anaemia [33]

David Cella and colleagues in Chicago have devised a core questionnaire called the FACT-G (Functional Assessment of Cancer Therapy-General) [66]. The 27 questions relate to the four dimensions of quality of life: physical, func-tional, emotional and social well-being. The measure is widely used to assess quality of life. This core questionnaire, developed in 1993, follows the same principles of the EORTC modular approach, whereby a number of additional scales can be added. In the case of studying patients with fatigue, a subscale called the FACT-F (Fatigue) with 13 items was created in 1997. A scale to as-sess anaemic patients, the FACT-An subscale, consists of a total of 47 questions, composed of the FACT-F with seven additional questions relating to conse-quences of anaemia other than fatigue [33]. Thus, the FACT-F contains items dealing with weakness, listlessness, need for sleep and tiredness that imposes limits on activity. The scale has highly reliable internal consistency (r = 0.95), making the fatigue subscale suitable for individual use. Among the additional questions in FACT-An are items dealing with light-headedness, headache and shortness of breath.

The development of both measures involved patients and health care pro-fessionals and the psychometric properties were assessed in a population of 50 mixed cancer patients in the US. The FACT-F demonstrated significant test-retest scores (alpha = 0.93), indicating that the scale could function indepen-dently as a single fatigue measure. The FACT-F also showed evidence of signif-icant correlation coefficients with other measures used to assess fatigue, i.e. POMS and Piper Fatigue Scale. There is evidence that FACT-F can discrimi-nate between levels of performance status, and that the scales successfully dis-criminate between patients who are anaemic and those who are not: patients with haemoglobin levels greater than 12 g/dl report significantly less fatigue and fewer non-fatigue symptoms of anaemia than those with haemoglobin values of 12 g/dl or less. In a recent study by Littlewood et al. [64] 359 chemotherapy patients were randomised to receive placebo or epoetin. Fatigue scores improved over the treatment period in the epoetin group, but worsened among patients receiving the placebo; the same was true for the non-fatigue, anaemia-related items on the FACT-An scale. The FACT-F and FACT-An scales have been translated into 25 languages. There is evidence that patients find the FACT-An scale easy to complete in about 10 minutes, although recent use with 2237 anaemic patients suggests that nine items had 3% or less missing data, seven items between 3% and 5% missing data, and two items up to 10% missing data [65]. Richardson [1] said that both the FACT-F and the FACT-An scales are relatively new and have not been subjected to extensive testing.

Conclusions

It is clear that for cancer patients fatigue is a significant problem, with an increase in recent years of measures to assess the condition. This review demonstrates that there are a number of key psychometric issues in the assessment of fatigue to ensure meaningful results. However, not every fatigue measure reviewed meets all challenging criteria. Many of the measures exhibit differing definitions of fatigue, and in some cases none at all, upon which to base the development of measuring tools. Frequently, there is no specific theory or plan to guide the development of the tool.

While many of the fatigue measures reported have both strengths and limitations, no blanket recommendation can be made as to which measure is more appropriate; it depends on the setting the clinician or researcher intends to use. It is clear that in certain circumstances one measure may be more appropriate than another; for example, when a detailed assessment of the social and the physical consequences of fatigue are required, a single, unidimensional tool such as the FACT-F (for individuals) or the EORTC QLQ-C30 fatigue scales (for groups) would not be ideal. However, when a simple indication of fatigue is needed, the two tools would possibly be useful measures.

There is a trade-off between efficiency and multidimensionality in clinical practice. Schneider [40] argues that in the present climate of clinical oncology many professionals could benefit from a brief 4- or 5-item measure that is valid in assessing fatigue, even in a general sense. However, it is clear from this discussion that no standard fatigue-measuring tool is used with cancer patients. While many new tools have been created in the last five years, more research on the function and value of the newer measures needs to be undertaken. Clinicians need to take great care in selecting instruments to measure fatigue, noting the most appropriate psychometric properties and, importantly, ensuring that the measure selected is appropriate for the task in hand.

References

1   Richardson A. Measuring fatigue in patients with cancer. Support Care Cancer 1998; 6: 94-100

2   Llewelyn MB. Assessing the fatigued patient. Br J Hosp Med 1996; 55: 125-9

3   Varricchio CG. Selecting a tool for measuring fatigue. Oncol Nurs Forum 1985; 12: 122-7

4   Winningham ML, Nail LM, Burke MB. Fatigue and the cancer experience: the state of knowledge. Oncol Nurs Forum 1994; 21: 23-36

5   Schwartz AL. The Schwartz Cancer Fatigue Scale: testing reliability and validity. Oncol Nurs Forum 1998; 25: 711-7

6   Barrere C, Trotta P, Foster J. The experience of fatigue in women undergoing radiation therapy for early stage breast cancer (abstract). Oncol Nurs Forum 1993; 20: 335

7   Ferrell B, Grant M, Dean G, Funk B, Ly J. "Bone tired": the experience of fatigue and its impact on quality of life. Oncol Nurs Forum 1996; 23: 1539-47

8   Glaus A, Crow R, Hammond S. A qualitative study to explore the concept of fatigue/tiredness in cancer patients and in healthy individuals. Support Care Cancer 1996; 4: 82-96

9   Haylock P, Hart L. Fatigue in patients receiving localised radiation. Cancer Nurs 1979; 2: 461-7

10   Jensen S, Given B. Fatigue affecting family caregivers of cancer patient. Cancer Nurs 1991; 14: 181-7

11   Smets E, Garssen B, De Haes JCJM. Application of the multidimensional fatigue inventory in cancer patients receiving radiotherapy. Br J Cancer 1996; 73: 241-5

12   Dimeo F, Stieglitz RD, Novelli-Fischer U, Fetscher S, Mertelsman R, Keul J. Correlation between physical performance and fatigue in cancer patients. Ann Oncol 1997; 8: 1251-5

13   Smets EMA, Visser MRM, Willems-Groot AFMN, et al. Fatigue and radiotherapy: (A) experience in patients undergoing treatment. Br J Cancer 1998; 78: 899-906

14   Okuyama T, Akechi T, Kugaya A, et al. Factors correlated with fatigue in disease-free breast cancer patients: application of the Cancer Fatigue Scale. Support Care Cancer 2000; 8: 215-22

15   Stone P, Richards M, Hardy J. Fatigue in patients with cancer. Eur J Cancer 1998; 34: 1670-6

16   Berglund G, Boland C, Fornandes T, et al. Late effects of adjuvant chemotherapy and postoperative radiotherapy on quality of life among breast cancer patients. Eur J Cancer 1991; 27: 1075-81

17   Simon AM, Zittoun R. Fatigue in cancer patients. Curr Opin Oncol 1999; 11: 244-9

18   Miaskowski C, Lee KA. Pain, fatigue, and sleep disturbances in oncology outpatients receiving radiation therapy for bone metastasis: a pilot study. J Pain Symptom Manage 1999; 17: 320-32

19   Hann DM, Garovoy N, Finkelstein B, Jacobsen PB, Azzarello LM, Fields KK. Fatigue and quality of life in breast cancer patients undergoing autologous stem cell transplantation: a longitudinal comparative study. J Pain Symptom Manage 1999; 17: 311-9

20   Jacobsen PB, Hann DM, Azzarello LM, Horton J, Balducci L, Lyman GH. Fatigue in women receiving adjuvant chemotherapy for breast cancer: characteristics, course, and correlates. J Pain Symptom Manage 1999; 18: 233-42

21   Beller E, Tattersall M, Lumley T, et al. Improved quality of life with megestrol acetate in patients with endocrine-insensitive advanced cancer: a randomised placebo-controlled trial. Australasian Megestrol Acetate Cooperative Study Group. Ann Oncol 1997; 8: 277-83

22   Ream E, Richardson A. From theory to practice: designing interventions to reduce fatigue in patients with cancer. Oncol Nurs Forum 1999; 26: 1295-303

23 Smets EMA, Visser MRM, Willems-Groot AFMN, Garssen B, Schuster-Uitterhoeve ALJ, de Haes JCJM. Fatigue and radiotherapy: (B) experience in patients 9 months following treatment. Br J Cancer 1998; 78: 907-12

24 Dimeo FC, Stieglitz RD, Novelli-Fischer U, Fetscher S, Keul J. Effects of physical activity on the fatiuge and psychologic status of cancer patients during chemotherapy. Cancer 1999; 85: 2273-7

25 Trijsburg R, van Knippenberg F, Rijpma S. Effects of psychological treatment on cancer patients: a critical review. Psychosomatic Medicine 1992; 54: 489-517

26 Telch C, Telch M. Group coping skills instruction and supportive group therapy for cancer patients: a comparison of strategies. J Consult Clin Psychol 1986; 54: 802-8

27 Bjordal K, Kaasa S, Mastekaasa A. Quality of life in patients treated for head and neck cancer: a follow-up study 7 to 11 years after radiotherapy. Int J Radiat Oncol Biol Phys 1994; 28: 847-56

28 Richardson A. Fatigue in cancer patients: a review of the literature Eur J Cancer 1995; 4: 20-32

29 Richardson A, Ream EK. Self-care behaviours initiated by chemotherapy patients in response to fatigue. Int J Nurs Stud 1997; 34: 35-43

30 Sneeuw KC, Aaronson NK, Osoba D, et al. The use of significant others as proxy raters of the quality of life of patients with brain cancer. Med Care 1997; 35: 490-506

31 Piper BF, Dibble SL, Dodd MJ, Weiss MC, Slaughter RE, Paul SM. The revised Piper Fatigue Scale: Psychometric evaluation in women with breast cancer. Oncol Nurs Forum 1998; 25: 677-84

32 Chalder T, Berelowitz G, Pawlikowska T, et al. Development of a fatigue scale. J Psychosom Res 1993; 37: 147-53

33 Cella D. The Functional Assessment of Cancer Therapy-Anemia (FACT-An) Scale: A new tool for the assessment of outcomes in cancer anemia and fatigue. Semin Hematol 1997; 34: 13-9

34 Hann DM, Jacobsen PB, Azzarello LM, et al. Measurement of fatigue in cancer patients: development and validation of the Fatigue Symptom Inventory. Qual Life Res 1998; 7: 301-10

35 Fayers PM, Machin D. Quality of life: assessment, analysis and interpretation. Chichester: John Wiley & Sons, 2000

36 Perneger TV, Leplege A, Etter JF. Cross-cultural adaptation of a psychometric instrument: two methods compared. J Clin Epidemiol 1999; 52: 1037-46

37 Bullinger M, Alonso J, Apolone G, et al. Translating health status questionnaires and evaluating their quality: the IQOLA Project approach. International Quality of Life Assessment. J Clin Epidemiol 1998; 51: 913-23

38 Wagner AK, Gandek B, Aaronson NK, et al. Cross-cultural comparisons of the content of SF-36 translations across 10 countries: results from the IQOLA Project. International Quality of Life Assessment. J Clin Epidemiol 1998; 51: 925-32

39 Rhoten D. Fatigue and the post-surgical patient. In: Norris CM, ed. Concept clarification in nursing. Rockville, MD: Aspen Publishers Inc, 1982; 277-300

40 Schneider RA. Reliability and validity of the Multidimensional Fatigue Inventory (MFI-20) and the Rhoten Fatigue Scale among rural cancer outpatients. Cancer Nursing 1998; 21: 370-3

41 Jacobsen PB, Stein K. Is fatigue a long-term side effect of breast cancer treatment? Cancer Control 1999; 6: 256-63

42 Piper BF, Lindsey AM, Dodd MJ, Ferketich S, Paul SM, Weller S. The development of an instrument to measure the subjective dimension of fatigue. In: Funk SG, Tournquist EM, Champagne MT, Copp LA, Weise RA, eds. Key aspects of comfort: management of pain, fatigue, and nausea. New York: Springer Verlag, 1989; 199-208

43 McNair DM, Lorr M, Dropplemann LF. The manual for the Profile of Mood States. San Diego, CA: Educational and Industrial Testing Service, 1971

44 Dean G, Spears L, Ferrell B, et al. Fatigue in patients with cancer receiving interferon alpha. Cancer Prac 1995; 3: 164-73

45 Smets EMA, Garssen ALJ, Schuster-Uitterhoeve ALJ, de Haes JCJM. Fatigue in cancer patients. Br J Cancer 1993; 68: 220-4

46 Pearson PG, Byars GE. The development and validation of a checklist measuring subjective fatigue. (Report no. 56-115). School of Aviation, USAF, Randolf AFB, Texas 1956

47 Smets EM, Garssen B, Bonke B, De Haes JCJM. The multidimensional fatigue inventory (MFI). Psychometric qualities of an instrument to assess fatigue. J Psychosom Res 1995; 39: 315-25

48 Mendoza TR, Wang XS, Cleeland CS, et al. The rapid assessment of fatigue severity in cancer patients: use of the Brief Fatigue Inventory. Cancer 1999; 85: 1186-96

49 Schwartz AL. Fatigue mediates the effects of exercise on quality of life. Qual Life Res 1999; 8: 529-38

50 Glaus A. Assessment of fatigue in cancer and non-cancer patients and in healthy individuals. Support Care Cancer 1993; 1: 305-15

51 Blesch KS, Paice JA, Wickham R, et al. Correlates of fatigue in people with breast or lung cancer. Oncol Nurs Forum 1991; 18: 81-7

52 Ware JE, Sherbourne CD. The MOS 36-Item Short-Form Health Survey (SF-36): I. Conceptual framework and item selection. Med Care 1992; 30: 473-81

53 Andrykowski MA, Curran SL, Lightner R. Off-treatment fatigue in breast cancer survivors: a controlled comparison. J Behav Med 1998 21: 1-18

54 Bower JE, Ganz PA, Desmond KA, Rowland JH, Meyerowitz BE, Belin TR. Fatigue in breast cancer survivors: occurrence, correlates, and impact of quality of life. J Clin Oncol 2000; 18: 743-53

55 Brazier JE, Walters SJ, Nicholl JP, Kohler B. Using the SF-36 and Euroqol on an elderly population. Qual Life Res 1996; 5: 195-204

56 Lyons RA, Wareham K, Lucas M, Price D, Williams J, Hutchins HA. SF-36 scores vary by method of administration: implications for study design. J Public Health Med 1999; 21: 41-5

57 Fayers PM, Machin D. Summarizing quality of life data using graphical methods. In: Staquet MJ, Hays RD, Fayers PM, eds. Quality of life assessment in clinical trials: Methods and practice. Oxford Medical Publications, 1998

58 Glimelius B, Linne T, Hoffman K, et al. Epoetin beta in the treament of anemia in patients with advanced gastrointestinal cancer. J Clin Oncol 1998; 16: 434-40

59 Sprangers MAG, Van Dam FSAM, Broersen J, et al. Revealing response shift in longitudinal research on fatigue: the use of the Thentest Approach. Acta Oncol 1999; 38: 709-18

60 Pater JL, Zee B, Palmer M, Johnston D, Osoba D. Fatigue in patients with cancer: results with National Cancer Institute of Canada Clinical Trials Group studies employing the EORTC QLQ-C30. Support Care Cancer 1997; 5: 410-3

61 Carlsson M, Strang P, Bjurstrom C. Treatment modality affects long-term quality of life in gynaecological cancer. Anticancer Res 2000; 20: 563-8

62 Blazeby JM, Brookes ST, Alderson D. Prognostic value of quality of life scores in patients with oesophageal cancer. Br J Surg 2000; 87: 362-73

63 Giaccone G, Splinter TA, Debruyne C, et al. Randomized study of paclitaxel-cisplatin versus cisplatin-teniposide in patients with advanced non-small-cell lung cancer. The European Organization for Research and Treatment of Cancer Lung Cooperative Group. J Clin Oncol 1998; 16: 2133-41

64 Littlewood TJ, Bajetta E, Cella D, Evanston H. Efficacy and quality of life outcomes of epoetin alfa in a double-blind, placebo-controlled multicenter study of cancer patients receiving non-platinum containing chemotherapy. Proc ASCO 1999; 18: 574a

65 Demetri GD, Kris M, Wade J, Degos L, Cella D. Quality-of-life benefit in chemotherapy patients treated with epoetin alfa is independent of disease response or tumor type: results from a prospective community oncology study. J Clin Oncol 1998; 16: 3412-25
66 Yellen SB, Cella DF, Webster K, Blendowski C, Kaplan E. Measuring fatigue and other anemia-related symptoms with the Functional Assessment of Cancer Therapy (FACT) measurement system. J Pain Symptom Manage 1997 13: 63-74

ESO Scientific Updates, Vol. 5
Fatigue and Cancer
M. Marty and S. Pecorelli, editors
© 2001 Elsevier Science B.V. All rights reserved

Epoetin Alfa Intervention for Anemia-Related Fatigue in Cancer Patients

Loretta M. Itri

Clinical Affairs, Ortho Biotech Products, L.P., Raritan, NJ, USA

Introduction

Anemia is common in cancer patients and may have a complex symptomatology and etiology [1]. Fatigue is the hallmark symptom of anemia; other signs/ symptoms include myriad cardiovascular and neurologic manifestations of decreased tissue oxygenation, such as dizziness, chest pain, shortness of breath, headache, and impaired cognitive function [2]. Cancer-related anemia may stem from disease-related processes, such as iron or nutritional deficiencies, hemolysis, bone marrow infiltration, and/or long-standing blood loss. Anemia of chronic disease (i.e. low serum iron and total iron-binding capacity, bone marrow erythroid hypoplasia, inappropriately low serum erythropoietin levels) often accompanies a diagnosis of cancer, with subsequent exacerbation during myelotoxic chemotherapy, radiation therapy, or chemoradiation regimens [1].

The risk of chemotherapy-induced anemia is dependent on the type and intensity of the current regimen and the patient's previous history of myelosuppressive therapies. A recent retrospective review of the incidence of chemotherapy-induced anemia revealed a high incidence of mild-to-moderate anemia with numerous single-agent and combination regimens used in the treatment of solid tumors and nonmyeloid malignancies [1]. First-line treatment of many solid tumors (e.g. advanced non-small cell lung and ovarian cancers) includes platinum-based chemotherapy, which is known to be highly myelotoxic. In addition, newer antineoplastic agents, such as taxanes (paclitaxel, docetaxel), gemcitabine, vinorelbine, and topoisomerase-I inhibitors (topotecan, irinotecan) have been shown to cause anemia in a substantial proportion of patients [1]. The myelotoxic potential of radiation therapy also is well recognized, but documentation of anemia in the radiation oncology setting has been limited. An ongoing retrospective study at Beth Israel Medical Center in New York has shown that there is a high incidence of mild-to-moderate anemia (hemoglobin [Hb]

Address for correspondence: L.M. Itri, Ortho Biotech Products, L.P., Clinical Affairs, 700 US Highway 202, Raritan, NJ 08869-0670, USA. Tel.: +1-908-7044509, fax: +1-908-2530434, e-mail: Litri@obius.jnj.com

levels 10-12 g/dl) at the initiation and completion of radiation therapy [3]. Based on preliminary findings, 32% of male patients and 57% of female patients were anemic (Hb level <12 g/dl) at presentation for radiation therapy. At completion of radiation therapy, anemia was present in 51% and 64% of male and female patients, respectively. The incidence of anemia at completion of radiation therapy ranged from 32% (prostate cancer patients) to 82% (uterine-cervix cancer patients) [3].

Fatigue that commonly accompanies cancer is highly debilitating and exerts a significant negative impact on quality of life (QOL) [4-6]. Cella and colleagues found that fatigue was the most frequent symptom in more than 1000 cancer and HIV patients (reported in 73% of patients), with a higher prevalence than pain (60%), anxiety (59%), sadness (58%), and nausea (30%) [7]. Recent surveys by the Fatigue Coalition (a multidisciplinary group of clinicians, researchers, and patient advocates; see also the chapter by G. Curt in this volume) explored the impact of fatigue on cancer patients who underwent chemotherapy alone or with radiation therapy and captured oncologists' perceptions of fatigue [4,6,8,9]. In the first survey, most of the patients (75%) suffered from fatigue, and one third indicated that they experienced fatigue on a daily basis [6]. This survey corroborated earlier reports that cancer-related fatigue occurs frequently and has significant debilitating effects. The Fatigue Coalition's second survey further extended the investigation of cancer-related fatigue, probing the physical, emotional, social, and economic impact of fatigue on cancer patients [4,8]. Most patients (76%) reported experiencing fatigue at least monthly, and approximately 50% of patients perceived the impact of fatigue to be significant. Cancer-related fatigue had important economic implications. More than three quarters of those surveyed reported that they missed at least one day of work per month or changed their employment status as the result of fatigue. Patients missed an average of 4.2 days of work per month, and many took unpaid family or medical leave (11%), discontinued working (28%), or went on disability (23%) [8]. This survey found that 40% of patients were not offered any recommendations to alleviate fatigue, and that bed rest/relaxation was the most common recommendation (37%). Only 9% of physicians recommended prescription medications to manage fatigue. A complete report of the results of the Fatigue Coalition's second survey is in press.

It is difficult to pinpoint the exact cause of fatigue in cancer patients [5]; however, the impact of chronic anemia on energy levels and the ability to perform daily activities has become more appreciated [7]. Until recently, patients with "physiologic" anemia (Hb level <8 g/dl or severe symptoms) were considered the most appropriate candidates for anemia management because of the risk of cardiovascular compromise [1,10,11]. This practice, however, does not give sufficient consideration to QOL or rehabilitation of patients [10]. In a continually evolving pattern of health care practices, increasing emphasis is being placed on QOL. Thus, clinicians are becoming more apt to treat "functional" anemia (Hb levels 10-12 g/dl), which may not be life-threatening but can impair QOL [11]. Transfusion may be warranted in patients who have extremely low Hb levels or exhibit pronounced symptoms; however, the inherent risks and shortcomings of transfusion, such as infection risks and supply/cost issues, make it a less than ideal method for treating mild-to-moderate anemia. Recombinant human erythropoietin (rHuEPO, epoetin alfa) was developed to provide a novel alternative to red blood cell (RBC) transfusion for treatment of cancer-related anemia [9].

Role of erythropoietin in cancer-related anemia

Erythropoietin is a glycoprotein that is produced primarily in the kidney (and, to a small extent [~5%], in the liver) [12,13]. Erythropoietin stimulates the growth, survival, and differentiation of erythroid progenitor cells [14]. Although their importance is unknown, erythropoietin receptors are found on a variety of nonerythroid cell types, including pluripotent hematopoietic progenitor cells, endothelial cells, neural crest cells, and embryonal stem cells. Biosynthesis of endogenous erythropoietin is regulated, at least in part, through a response to hypoxic conditions [15,16]. In fact, a thousandfold increase in erythropoietin may occur when oxygen availability is reduced [17-19].

An inverse correlation between Hb levels and erythropoietin concentrations characterizes anemia that results from some pathologic conditions. This correlation does not apply to patients with chronic renal failure, as production of erythropoietin is severely impaired or absent. Early studies that sought to elucidate the role of erythropoietin levels in cancer-related anemia were inconclusive. To better characterize cancer-related anemia, a study was conducted in which serum erythropoietin concentrations were determined by radioimmunoassay in 81 anemic (Hb level ≤12 g/dl) patients with solid tumors [20]. A control group included 24 men and women with iron-deficiency anemia. The mean Hb level was not significantly different between cancer patients and the control group (10.3 g/dl versus 9.8 g/dl); however, the mean serum immunoreactive erythropoietin level was significantly lower in cancer patients (33.4 U/L versus 76.6 U/L; p=0.001). A significant inverse linear correlation was observed between Hb levels and erythropoietin concentrations in the control group but not in the cancer patients. The blunted erythropoietin response observed in these solid tumor patients was consistent with the findings of some earlier studies. Overall, inadequate erythropoietin production appears to be an important contributing factor to the development of cancer-related anemia.

Historical overview of epoetin alfa for correcting anemia

Chronic renal failure experience

In early studies epoetin alfa demonstrated the ability to stimulate erythropoiesis in predialysis patients and those with end-stage renal disease (ESRD)

[21-24]. A phase I/II study of epoetin alfa 1.5 to 500 U/kg intravenously (IV) three times weekly (TIW) was conducted in patients with ESRD [23]. Dose-dependent increases in erythropoiesis were observed in patients receiving epoetin alfa 15 to 500 U/kg, and hematocrit increases of up to 10% within three weeks were demonstrated at the 500 U/kg dose level. The effectiveness and safety of epoetin alfa 150 or 300 U/kg IV TIW were further explored in a phase III multicenter study that enrolled 333 hemodialysis patients with hematocrit values ≤30% [21]. Within 18 weeks an increase in hematocrit occurred in 97.4% of patients, and RBC transfusions were eliminated in virtually all patients within two months of therapy. Overall, epoetin alfa has been established as an extremely successful treatment for anemia in patients with all stages of chronic renal failure. An extensive body of evidence also supports the QOL benefits of epoetin alfa in patients with chronic renal failure, including but not limited to improved energy/activity levels, sleeping/eating behavior, and sense of well-being [25].

HIV/AIDS experience

Anemia in HIV/AIDS patients may be related to underlying disease or medications, and zidovudine is frequently implicated as a therapy-related cause of anemia [26]. Placebo-controlled studies have shown that epoetin alfa TIW corrects anemia and reduces transfusion requirements in HIV/AIDS patients receiving zidovudine. These hematopoietic benefits appear to be most pronounced in patients with baseline serum erythropoietin levels ≤500 mU/ml [26,27]. More recently, epoetin alfa has produced significant hematopoietic improvements in patients receiving protease inhibitors.

Early studies in cancer patients

An early series of randomized, placebo-controlled studies evaluated the effects of epoetin alfa in three populations of cancer patients: those not receiving concomitant chemotherapy or radiotherapy, those receiving non-cisplatin-containing cyclic chemotherapy, and those receiving cisplatin-containing cyclic chemotherapy [28]. Patients who did not undergo chemotherapy received placebo or epoetin alfa 100 U/kg subcutaneously (SC) TIW for eight weeks, whereas patients who underwent chemotherapy received placebo or epoetin alfa 150 U/kg SC TIW for 12 weeks. The primary efficacy variables were hematocrit concentrations and transfusion requirements. Additional efficacy measures included the proportion of patients with resolution of anemia (i.e. attainment of hematocrit of ≥38% unrelated to transfusion) and response to therapy (i.e. increase in hematocrit of ≥6% unrelated to transfusion). Assessment of functional capacity (energy level, ability to perform daily activities, and overall QOL) was performed using a 100-mm linear analog scale assessment (LASA, also known as CLAS, cancer linear analog scale) prior to and at the end of treatment. Lower LASA scores represent less favorable patient self-reported perceptions of these parameters. A change in LASA score of approximately 10 mm generally is considered clinically meaningful.

Statistically significant (p<0.004) increases in hematocrit were observed with epoetin alfa compared with placebo (Table 1) in patients not receiving chemotherapy (n=118), as well as in patients receiving cisplatin-containing chemotherapy (n=124) or non-cisplatin-containing chemotherapy (n=153) [28]. Significantly greater proportions (p≤0.008) of patients receiving epoetin alfa achieved correction of anemia and response to therapy. A significant reduction in the percent of patients requiring transfusion was also observed. In a combined analysis of the two chemotherapy-treated groups, the percent of patients requiring transfusion at months 2 and 3 was significantly lower in the epoetin alfa group compared with the placebo group (27.8% versus 45.5%; p<0.005). QOL benefits of epoetin alfa were demonstrated, as epoetin alfa-treated patients with an increase in hematocrit of >6% achieved statistically significant (p<0.05) improvements in energy level, ability to perform daily activities, and overall QOL compared with the placebo group. An equivalent epoetin alfa response was reported for patients with hematologic or solid tumors, and treatment was well tolerated.

Table 1. Response to epoetin alfa in anemic cancer patients treated with or without chemotherapy [28]

		Hematocrit (%)		
	No.	Baseline	Final	Change
Non-chemotherapy				
Epoetin alfa	63	29.3	32.1	2.8*
Placebo	55	27.6	27.5	-0.1
Non-cisplatin chemotherapy				
Epoetin alfa	79	28.6	35.5	6.9*
Placebo	74	29.4	30.5	1.1
Cisplatin-containing chemotherapy				
Epoetin alfa	63	29.4	35.4	6.0*
Placebo	61	28.4	29.7	1.3

*p<0.004 versus placebo.

Recent clinical experience with epoetin alfa TIW therapy

More recently, treatment of chemotherapy-related anemia with epoetin alfa TIW was investigated in large-scale studies by the Procrit Study Groups and the European Epoetin Alfa Study Group (EEASG) (Table 2) [29-31]. All patients in these three studies were at least 18 years of age and were receiving chemotherapy for nonmyeloid malignancies. Only patients receiving non-cisplatin-containing chemotherapy were eligible to participate in the EEASG study [31]. Exclusion criteria that applied to all studies included uncontrolled hypertension or anemia that was attributable to other factors (e.g. iron, folate or vitamin B12 deficiencies) [29-31].

Measurement of QOL in all of these studies included a 100-mm LASA to assess energy level, ability to perform daily activities, and overall QOL. In addition, Functional Assessment of Cancer Therapy (FACT) questionnaires were used in the more recent studies. The FACT measurement system includes over 250 questions addressing health-related QOL in patients with chronic diseases [32]. The core FACT-General (FACT-G) questionnaire is useful in evaluating physical, functional, emotional, and social well-being in cancer patients. The FACT-Fatigue (FACT-F) and Fact-Anemia (FACT-An) instruments were produced by adding fatigue and anemia-focused questions (Fatigue Subscale and Anemia Subscale) to the FACT-G scale (Fig. 1) [2,32]. The FACT-An is the QOL assessment tool most frequently used in clinical studies of cooperative oncology groups.

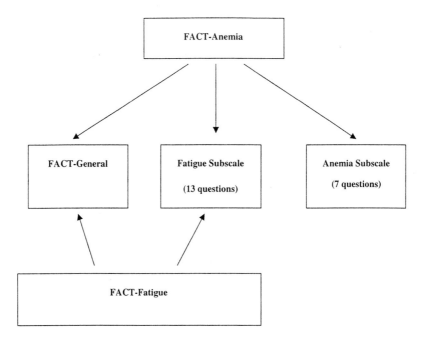

Fig. 1. The functional assessment of cancer therapy (FACT) measurement system [2,32].

Table 2. Phase III and IV clinical studies of epoetin alfa TIW for cancer-related anemia [29-31]

Study (phase)	Duration	Study design	Patient criteria	Dosage regimen
Glaspy et al. 1997 [30] (Phase IV)	16 wk	• Open-label • Nonrandomized • Noncomparative • Multicenter (US)	• Nonmyeloid malignancy • CT (with or without platinum) • Life expectancy ≥6 mo • Diagnosis of anemia	Epoetin alfa 150 U/kg SC TIW; if inadequate response after 8 wks, increase to 300 U/kg TIW
Demetri et al 1998 [29] (Phase IV)	16 wk	• Open-label • Nonrandomized • Noncomparative • Multicenter (US)	• Nonmyeloid malignancy • CT (with or without platinum) • Life expectancy ≥6 mo • Hb ≤11 g/dl	Epoetin alfa 10,000 U SC TIW; if increase in Hb <1 g/dl after 4 wks, increase to 20,000 U TIW; if increase in Hb <1 g/dl after an additional 4 wks, discontinue
EEASG 1999 [31] (Phase III)	16-28 wk	• Randomized • Double-blind • Placebo-controlled • Multicenter • Multinational (Europe)	• Nonmyeloid malignancy • Non-platinum CT • ECOG PS ≤3 • Life expectancy ≥6 mo • Hb ≤10.5 g/dl or 1.5 g/dl decrease during CT (per cycle or per mo) with Hb ≤12 g/dl at enrollment	Epoetin alfa 150 U/kg (or placebo) SC TIW plus supplemental iron; if Hb rise <1g/dl or reticulocyte increase <40,000/μl after 4 wks, increase to 300 U/kg SC TIW for a total of 12-24 wks (or 3-6 CT cycles) plus 4 wks post-CT

TIW = three times weekly; EEASG = European Epoetin Alfa Study Group; SC = subcutaneously; CT = chemotherapy; Hb = hemoglobin; ECOG = Eastern Cooperative Oncology Group; PS = performance status; HCT = hematocrit

Procrit* Study Group experience

Initial phase IV study [30]

In the first of two phase IV, open-label, community-based, multicenter studies, 2342 anemic (undefined Hb level) patients undergoing chemotherapy for non-myeloid malignancies received epoetin alfa 150 U/kg SC TIW for up to 16 weeks [30]. A dosage increase to 300 U/kg TIW was permitted after eight weeks of therapy if response was suboptimal. Assessments performed at monthly clinic visits included Hb and hematocrit, blood pressure, transfusion requirements, and adverse events. Effects of epoetin alfa on QOL were measured via the LASA parameters used in the placebo-controlled studies by Abels et al.: energy level, ability to perform daily activities, and overall QOL. Changes in LASA scores were analyzed by measures of statistical significance and effect sizes, which provide an estimate of the clinical relevance of observed changes (small but significant effect size: 0.20; medium effect size: 0.50; large effect size: 0.80) [30]. This study also included a retrospective collection of tumor response data to evaluate the possible impact of disease response on QOL; tumor response data were available for 759 patients.

The evaluable population consisted of 2030 of the 2342 enrolled patients. Most of the evaluable patients (77%) had solid tumors, with the following distribution: lung (22%), breast (18%), gynecologic (14%), gastrointestinal (6%), prostate (4%), head/neck (2%), bladder (2%), pancreas, esophagus, and renal (1% each), and other cancers (6%). Hematologic malignancies represented the remainder of the population (23%). Chemotherapeutic regimens administered during the study period consisted of a variety of cisplatin-containing regimens (22%), carboplatin-containing regimens (18%), or non-platinum-based regimens (60%). The mean baseline Hb level was 9.2 g/dl. During the month before study entry, 21.9% of patients had received a RBC transfusion, with a mean number of 0.57 units per patient. Mean baseline LASA scores were <50 mm, indicating that patients perceived substantial impairment in energy level, ability to perform daily activities, and overall QOL.

During the four-month treatment period, the mean Hb level increased progressively; increases from baseline to each monthly visit were statistically significant ($p<0.001$) [30]. An overall 1.8 g/dl increase in Hb level to a mean of 11.0 g/dl was observed in 2019 patients with both baseline and final Hb measurements ($p<0.001$ versus baseline). A Hb level increase of ≥2.0 g/dl was documented in 53.4% of patients who did not receive a transfusion during the study period. The mean number of patients requiring transfusion and the mean number of transfusions administered (per patient per month) were significantly reduced ($p<0.001$) after the first month of epoetin alfa treatment, with continued reductions during the study. Transfusions were required in 21.9% of evaluable pa-

---

* Epoetin alfa is marketed as Procrit® (Ortho Biotech Products, L.P., USA) and as Eprex®/Erypo® (Ortho Biotech/Janssen-Cilag, Europe).

tients during the first month, 14.8% of all patients during the second month, 10.7% of all patients during the third month, and 10.3% of all patients during the fourth month after initiation of epoetin alfa therapy.

Baseline and final LASA scores were available for 1498 patients [30]. Mean (percent) changes in energy level, ability to perform daily activities, and overall QOL were 15.0 mm (38%), 13.1 mm (32%), and 11.0 mm (24%), respectively. Furthermore, medium-to-large effects were observed for changes in energy level (39.4 mm to 54.4 mm, effect size of 0.70), ability to perform daily activities (40.8 mm to 53.9 mm, effect size of 0.55), and overall QOL (46.4 mm to 57.4 mm, effect size of 0.47). Significant improvements from baseline to final LASA scores occurred for all three parameters. In addition, the improvement in each of the LASA parameters was directly (r=0.27 to 0.30) and significantly (p<0.001) correlated with the magnitude of Hb level increase from baseline. Greater Hb level increases were associated with greater increases in mean LASA scores. However, significant (p<0.001) increases in mean energy level, ability to perform daily activities, and overall QOL scores were observed in patients with any positive change in Hb level. Retrospective analysis of tumor response data demonstrated that significant (p<0.05) increases in energy level occurred in all tumor response groups (i.e., progressive disease to complete remission). Statistically significant (p<0.05) improvements in the ability to perform daily activities and overall QOL were observed in patients with a complete response, partial response, or stable disease. In patients with progressive disease these parameters remained relatively unchanged from baseline to final evaluation. Epoetin alfa was well tolerated in this study [30] and subsequent studies by the Procrit Study Group and EEASG, and most reported adverse events were attributed to the underlying disease or concomitant chemotherapy [29-31].

Second phase IV study [29]

A second phase IV, open-label, community-based study was conducted to examine the effects of epoetin alfa in 2370 anemic cancer patients [29]. As in the earlier study, patients undergoing chemotherapy for nonmyeloid malignancies were eligible to receive a 16-week course of epoetin alfa. Patients were initially treated with epoetin alfa 10,000 U SC TIW. The dose was increased to 20,000 U SC TIW if the increase in Hb level was <1.0 g/dl after four weeks of therapy. This dose-titration schedule was more aggressive than that used in the earlier study. A positive hematopoietic response was defined as an increase in Hb level of ≥2 g/dl and/or achieving a Hb level of ≥12 g/dl. QOL assessments were completed by patients at baseline, before chemotherapy administration at month 2, and at study completion (month 4) or study withdrawal. QOL was evaluated with the FACT-An questionnaire and LASA of energy level, ability to perform daily activities, and overall QOL, allowing comparison with the results of the earlier study. An important feature of this study was that it prospectively addressed the influence of tumor response on QOL in anemic cancer patients treated with epoetin alfa [29].

The evaluable population was comprised of 2289 of the 2370 enrolled population (97%). As in the earlier study, most patients (78%) had solid tumors and 22% of patients had hematologic malignancies. Solid tumors included lung cancer (24%), breast cancer (17%), gynecologic cancer (13%), gastrointestinal cancer (9%), and other cancers (16%). Patients with all disease stages were enrolled to ensure that the study population was representative of community-based practice. Platinum-containing chemotherapy was administered to 1031 of the evaluable patients (45%), and approximately 10% of patients received chemotherapy plus radiation therapy. The mean baseline Hb level for all evaluable patients was 9.3 g/dl, and a total of 653 patients (29%) received transfusions during the previous month. All of the mean baseline LASA scores were less than 50 mm, indicating perceptions of functional and QOL impairment prior to initiation of epoetin alfa.

A positive response to treatment was achieved in 1406 of the evaluable patients (61%), and 74% of responding patients met both response criteria (increase in Hb level of ≥2 g/dl and attainment of a Hb level of ≥12 g/dl) [29]. A mean Hb level increase of 2.0 g/dl (to 11.3 g/dl) occurred from baseline to final evaluation (p<0.001) [29]. In 63% of patients Hb levels increased by >1.0 g/dl after four weeks of treatment. In addition, the overall percentage of patients requiring transfusion and the number of units transfused per patient decreased significantly (p<0.001) during the first month and continued to decrease throughout the study.

Total FACT-An and Anemia Subscale scores improved significantly (p<0.001) from baseline to final evaluation in patients with data from these assessments (n=1484) [29]. Patients with mean Hb level increases of ≥2 g/dl experienced the greatest positive increase in total FACT-An and Anemia Subscale scores. Mean (percent) improvements in LASA scores for energy level, ability to perform daily activities, and overall QOL were 11.5 mm (24%), 11.1 mm (28%), and 9.8 mm (21%), respectively; all of these changes were statistically significant (p<0.001). Increased Hb levels were associated with higher energy levels, ability to perform daily activities, and overall QOL scores. The correlation between increased overall QOL and increased Hb level was direct and significant (r=0.235; p<0.001) [29]. Tumor response analysis revealed that patients who had a complete/partial response or stable disease, but failed to attain a Hb response, did not achieve significant increases in LASA scores. Hb increases were directly and significantly (p<0.001) correlated with higher overall QOL scores in patients with a complete response, partial response, or stable disease. Patients with progressive disease experienced little change in QOL. This study confirmed that QOL improvements during epoetin alfa therapy are independent of disease response to anticancer therapy.

Incremental analysis of the Procrit Study Group studies

An incremental analysis of data from the phase IV Procrit Study Group studies of epoetin alfa TIW was conducted to identify the Hb level at which QOL is optimized [33]. Based on preliminary results, a statistically significant (p<0.01), nonlinear correlation exists between Hb level and QOL. The greatest increase in LASA and FACT-An scores (per unit change in Hb level) was achieved when the Hb level increased from 11 to 12 g/dl (range, 11 to 13 g/dl). Importantly, this finding was unaffected by controlling for the following variables: tumor type/status, transfusions, number of days on study, and extent of chemotherapy and radiotherapy. This analysis supports the perception that correcting mild-to-moderate anemia leads to QOL benefits in anemic patients receiving chemotherapy.

EEASG experience [31]

The effects of epoetin alfa TIW on Hb levels, transfusion requirements, and QOL were recently assessed in a placebo-controlled, double-blind study conducted by the EEASG [31]. Patients enrolled in this multinational study (n=375) received non-platinum-containing chemotherapy and were randomized to treatment with epoetin alfa 150 U/kg SC TIW (increased to 300 U/kg SC TIW at four weeks if response was inadequate) or placebo for a maximum of six chemotherapy cycles and four weeks postchemotherapy. Evaluation of QOL was conducted by 1) CLAS of energy level, ability to perform daily activities, and overall QOL; 2) the FACT-An, including the Fatigue and Anemia Subscales; 3) the FACT-G; and 4) the Medical Outcomes Study Short Form-36 (SF-36), one of the most utilized generic health status measures in the US and Europe.

Preliminary findings of this study were presented at the 35th Annual Meeting of the American Society of Clinical Oncology (ASCO) [31]. At baseline, the mean Hb level was 9.9 g/dl in the epoetin alfa group and 9.7 g/dl in the placebo group. The mean change in Hb level from baseline to end of study was 2.2 g/dl (to 12.1 g/dl) in the epoetin alfa group and 0.5 g/dl (to 10.2 g/dl) in the placebo group (p<0.001). A significant difference in the percentage of patients requiring transfusion from the end of week 4 to study completion was observed between the epoetin alfa and placebo groups (24.7% and 39.5%, respectively; p=0.006). Changes in LASA energy level score were +7.84 for epoetin alfa and -5.81 for placebo (p<0.001); changes in the ability to perform daily activities were +7.28 for epoetin alfa and -5.99 for placebo (p<0.01); changes in overall QOL scores were +4.55 for epoetin alfa and -5.97 for placebo (p<0.01). The epoetin alfa group achieved significant (p<0.05) improvements in mean FACT-G and FACT-An scores (Fatigue and Anemia Subscales) compared with the placebo group, which had decreased scores from baseline to final evaluation. Differences in the fatigue-related SF-36 questions were also demonstrated; mean SF-36 overall physical and mental QOL scores favored the epoetin alfa group, but the between-group difference did not reach statistical significance [31]. The results of this comparative European study were consistent with those of the phase IV US studies and confirmed, in a placebo-controlled setting, the efficacy of epoetin alfa TIW in increasing Hb levels, reducing transfusion requirements, and improving multiple aspects of QOL in patients receiving chemotherapy.

Clinical experience with once-weekly (QW) epoetin alfa therapy

The most recent community-based study investigated an epoetin alfa dosage regimen that would increase the convenience of therapy in oncology practice: 40,000 U SC QW, with the possibility of increasing the dosage to 60,000 U QW if Hb levels did not rise by ≥1 g/dl after four weeks of treatment [35]. Treatment continued for a maximum of 16 weeks and was temporarily discontinued in patients whose Hb level exceeded 13 g/dl (resumed when Hb was 12 g/dl, with gradual titration from 75% of the previous dose). The design of this study of epoetin alfa QW was similar to that of the studies of epoetin alfa TIW. Efficacy variables included Hb levels, transfusion requirements, and QOL scores (LASA and the Anemia Subscale of the FACT-An instrument). Safety was evaluated by monitoring adverse events.

A total of 2964 of 3012 enrolled patients have been evaluated [34]. Preliminary results were presented at the 35th Annual Meeting of ASCO [35]. The mean Hb level increased significantly from baseline to final evaluation (p<0.001). The percentage of patients receiving transfusions declined significantly (p<0.001), as did the number of units of RBC transfusions administered per month. At baseline all mean LASA scores were below 50 mm on the 100-mm scale, suggesting functional impairment. Significant increases in all three LASA parameters were achieved from baseline to final evaluation (p<0.05 for all changes). LASA overall QOL scores increased significantly (p<0.05) in all patients who achieved a Hb level increase. The magnitude of increase in Hb level was associated with the improvement observed in LASA overall QOL score. Mean (percent) increases in overall QOL scores were: 8.2 mm (17.2%) for Hb increases of 0 to 2 g/dl, 12.2 mm (25.2%) for Hb increases of >2 to 4 g/dl, and 15.4 mm (32.3%) for Hb increases of >4 g/dl [35].

A statistically significant improvement (p<0.05) in the Anemia Subscale of the FACT-An scores was observed from baseline to final evaluation. As with LASA, greater changes in the Anemia Subscale of the FACT-An scores were associated with greater changes in Hb level. Mean (percent) increases in the Anemia Subscale of the FACT-An scores were 4.8 (11.2%) for Hb level increases of 0 to 2 g/dl, 7.7 (17.6%) for Hb increases of >2 to 4 g/dl, and 11.0 (25.4%) for Hb level increases >4 g/dl. Treatment was well tolerated, and the vast majority of serious adverse events were considered to be unrelated to epoetin alfa therapy and were attributed to the underlying disease and/or chemotherapy. The efficacy and safety profiles of epoetin alfa QW were similar to those established for epoetin alfa TIW. This more convenient regimen has the ability to increase Hb levels, reduce transfusion requirements, and improve QOL in patients receiving chemotherapy.

Conclusion

An increased emphasis on QOL has resulted in a shift toward more frequent treatment of mild-to-moderate anemia, which may not be life-threatening but may affect QOL. As advancements in anticancer therapy result in survival gains, certain types of cancer may be regarded as chronic illnesses. Thus, mild-to-moderate anemia is often a long-term condition in the cancer population, requiring new approaches to treatment. Epoetin alfa, an alternative to blood transfusion in patients with anemia, is effective in improving Hb levels and transfusion requirements in patients actively receiving chemotherapy. In large-scale studies by the Procrit Study Groups and the EEASG, epoetin alfa therapy consistently improved hematopoietic (Hb levels, transfusion requirements) and QOL outcomes, as assessed by FACT questionnaires and LASA of energy levels, the ability to perform daily activities, and overall QOL. Epoetin alfa had the greatest impact on energy levels in these phase III and IV studies. Although cancer-related fatigue has substantial functional (both physical and psychological) and economic consequences, health care providers tend to overlook this condition [8]. A greater sensitivity to the problem of cancer-related fatigue is imperative. It is anticipated that the availability of treatment options that target underlying causes of cancer-related fatigue will improve prospects in this area. Broader application of epoetin alfa therapy has the potential to contribute to a reduction in the impact of anemia-related fatigue on cancer patients.

References

1   Groopman JE, Itri LM. Chemotherapy-induced anemia in adults: incidence and treatment. J Natl Cancer Inst 1999; 91: 1616-34
2   Cella D. Factors influencing quality of life in cancer patients: anemia and fatigue. Semin Oncol 1998; 25 (suppl 7): 43-6
3   Harrison LB, Shasha D, Shiaova L, White C, Ramdeen B, Portenoy R. Prevalence of anemia in cancer patients undergoing radiation therapy [abstract 1849]. Proc Am Soc Clin Oncol 2000; 19; 471a. Poster presentation at the Thirty-Sixth Annual Meeting of the American Society of Clinical Oncology, New Orleans, LA, May 20-23, 2000
4   Curt GA, Breitbart W, Cella DF, et al. Impact of cancer-related fatigue on the lives of patients [abstract 2214]. Proc Am Soc Clin Oncol 1999; 18: 573a
5   Portenoy RK, Itri LM. Cancer-related fatigue: guidelines for evaluation and management. Oncologist 1999; 4: 1-10
6   Vogelzang NJ, Breitbart W, Cella D, et al for the Fatigue Coalition. Patient, caregiver, and oncologist perceptions of cancer-related fatigue: results of a tripart assessment survey. Semin Hematol 1997; 34 (suppl 2): 4-12
7   Cella D, Mo F, Peterman A. Anemia, fatigue and quality of life in people with cancer and HIV infection [abstract 571]. Blood 1996; 88 (suppl 1): 146a
8   Curt GA. The impact of fatigue on patients with cancer: overview of FATIGUE 1 and 2. Oncologist 2000; 5 (suppl 2): 9-12
9   Itri LM. Optimal hemoglobin levels for cancer patients. Semin Oncol 2000; 27 (suppl 4): 12-15

10   Ludwig H, Fritz E. Anemia in cancer patients. Semin Oncol 1998; 25 (suppl 7): 2-6
11   Pecorelli S. Introduction: Suboptimal hemoglobin levels: do they impact patients and their therapy? Semin Oncol 2000; 27 (suppl 4): 1-3
12   Fried W. The liver as a source of extrarenal erythropoietin production. Blood 1972; 40: 671-7
13   Jacobson LO, Goldwasser E, Fried W, Plzak LF. Studies on erythropoiesis. VII. The role of the kidney in the production of erythropoietin. Trans Assoc Am Physicians 1957; 70: 305-17
14   Witthuhn BA, Quelle FW, Silvennoinen O, et al. JAK2 associates with the erythropoietin receptor and is tyrosine phosphorylated and activated following stimulation with erythropoietin. Cell 1993; 74: 227-36
15   Goldberg MA, Dunning SP, Bunn HF. Regulation of the erythropoietin gene: evidence that the oxygen sensor is a heme protein. Science 1988; 242: 1412-5
16   Goldberg MA, Glass GA, Cunningham JM, Bunn HF. The regulated expression of erythropoietin by two human hepatoma cell lines. Proc Natl Acad Sci USA 1987; 84: 7972-6
17   Eckardt K-U, Koury ST, Tan CC, et al. Distribution of erythropoietin producing cells in rat kidneys during hypoxic hypoxia. Kidney Int 1993; 43: 815-23
18   Koury ST, Koury MJ, Bondurant MC, Caro J, Graber SE. Quantitation of erythropoietin-producing cells in kidneys of mice by in situ hybridization: correlation with hematocrit, renal erythropoietin mRNA, and serum erythropoietin concentration. Blood 1989; 74: 645-51
19   Ratcliffe PJ. Molecular biology of erythropoietin. Kidney Int 1993; 44: 887-904
20   Miller CB, Jones RJ, Piantadosi S, Abeloff MD, Spivak JL. Decreased erythropoietin response in patients with the anemia of cancer. N Engl J Med 1990; 322: 1689-92
21   Eschbach JW, Abdulhadi MH, Browne JK, et al. Recombinant human erythropoietin in anemic patients with end-stage renal disease. Ann Intern Med 1989; 111: 992-1000
22   Eschbach JW, Kelly MR, Haley NR, Abels RI, Adamson JW. Treatment of the anemia of progressive renal failure with recombinant human erythropoietin. N Engl J Med 1989; 321: 158-63
23   Eschbach JW, Egrie JC, Downing MR, Browne JK, Adamson JW. Correction of the anemia of end-stage renal disease with recombinant human erythropoietin. N Engl J Med 1987; 316: 73-8
24   Winearls CG, Oliver DO, Pippard MJ, Reid C, Downing MR, Cotes PM. Effect of human erythropoietin derived from recombinant DNA on the anaemia of patients maintained by chronic haemodialysis. Lancet 1986; 2: 1175-8
25   Macdougall IC. Quality of life and anemia: the nephrology experience. Semin Oncol 1998; 25 (suppl 7): 39-42
26   Henry DH. Experience with epoetin alfa and acquired immunodeficiency syndrome anemia. Semin Oncol 1998; 25 (suppl 7): 64-8
27   Procrit® (epoetin alfa) prescribing information. Ortho Biotech, Inc., Raritan, NJ, October 1999
28   Abels RI. Recombinant human erythropoietin in the treatment of the anaemia of cancer. Acta Haematol 1992; 87 (suppl 1): 4-11
29   Demetri GD, Kris M, Wade J, Degos L, Cella D for the Procrit Study Group. Quality-of-life benefit in chemotherapy patients treated with epoetin alfa is independent of disease response or tumor type: results from a prospective community oncology study. J Clin Oncol 1998; 16: 3412-25
30   Glaspy J, Bukowski R, Steinberg D, Taylor C, Tchekmedyian S, Vadhan-Raj S for the Procrit Study Group. Impact of therapy with epoetin alfa on clinical outcomes in patients with nonmyeloid malignancies during cancer chemotherapy in community oncology practice. J Clin Oncol 1997; 15: 1218-34

31 Littlewood TJ, Bajetta E, Cella D for the European Epoetin Alfa Study Group. Efficacy and quality of life outcomes of epoetin alfa in a double-blind, placebo-controlled multicenter study of cancer patients receiving non-platinum containing chemotherapy [abstract 2217]. Proc Am Soc Clin Oncol 1999; 18: 574a. Presentation at the Thirty-Fifth Annual Meeting of the American Society of Clinical Oncology, Atlanta, GA, May 15-18, 1999

32 Yellen SB, Cella DF, Webster K, Blendowski C, Kaplan E. Measuring fatigue and other anemia-related symptoms with the Functional Assessment of Cancer Therapy (FACT) measurement system. J Pain Symptom Manage 1997; 13: 63-74

33 Cleeland CS, Demetri GD, Glaspy J, Cella DF et al. Identifying hemoglobin level for optimal quality of life: results of an incremental analysis [abstract 2215]. Proc Am Soc Clin Oncol 1999; 18: 574a

34 Gabrilove JL, Cleeland CS, Livingston RB, Sarokhan B, Winer E, Einhorn LH. Clinical evaluation of once-weekly dosing of epoetin alfa in chemotherapy patients: improvements in hemoglobin and quality of life are similar to three-times-weekly dosing. J Clin Oncol 2001; 19 (in press)

35 Gabrilove JL, Einhorn LH, Livingston RB, Winer E, Cleeland CS. Once-weekly dosing of epoetin alfa is similar to three-times-weekly dosing in increasing hemoglobin and quality of life [abstract 2216]. Proc Am Soc Clin Oncol 1999; 18: 574a. Presentation at the Thirty-Fifth Annual Meeting of the American Society of Clinical Oncology, Atlanta, GA, May 15-18, 1999

ESO Scientific Updates, Vol. 5
Fatigue and Cancer
M. Marty and S. Pecorelli, editors
© 2001 Elsevier Science B.V. All rights reserved

Depression and Cancer

Sylvie Dolbeault[1], Gilles Marx[2] and Pierre Saltel[3]

1   Psycho-Oncology Unit, Institut Curie, Paris
2   Psycho-Oncology Unit, Centre René Huguenin, Saint-Cloud
3   Psycho-Oncology Unit, Centre Léon Bérard, Lyon, France

Introduction

The problem of depression in cancer patients needs to be re-examined in light of the therapeutic progress made in the field of oncology, which has transformed the prognosis of this disease. Cancer is now a potentially curable, somatic disease with a chronic course. Cancers and the therapeutic strategies adopted to treat them constitute repeated stress for the patient and the family, but also for health care professionals. In addition to dealing with the patient's physical pain, the dimension of mental distress therefore becomes a major challenge that concerns all partners of the health care process. However, the concepts and methods designed to investigate the issue of psychological distress in oncology remain poorly defined and the diagnosis of depression in oncology and the modalities of its management are still controversial. The quality of the relational approach and the communication between the patient and the health care professionals will be decisive in terms of the quality of management and the satisfaction of the patient and his/her family.

Distress and depression

The most recent studies propose a pragmatic approach based on the concept of "psychological distress". Jimmie Holland [1] defines this concept as follows: "Distress is an unpleasant experience of an emotional, psychological, social, or spiritual nature that interferes with the ability to cope with cancer treatment. It extends along a continuum, from common, normal feelings of vulnerability, sadness and fear, to problems that are disabling, such as true depression, anxiety, panic, and the feeling of isolation or spiritual crisis".

Address for correspondence: S. Dolbeault, Psycho-Oncology Unit, Institut Curie,
26, rue d'Ulm, 75246 Paris cedex 05, France. Tel.: +33-1-44324033, fax: +33-1-44324017,
e-mail: sylvie.dolbeault@curie.net

The term was chosen because it is less stigmatising than others having a psychopathological connotation, and is more acceptable and easier to use for health care professionals who question the patient about his or her emotional state.

It should be noted that this approach is based on the one already applied to pain management and, like this method, can be used to demonstrate and quantify the patient's needs. It can define the various dimensions of the concept of psychological distress without stratifying its various aspects. This approach assumes the existence of a continuum of mental states ranging from "normal" to "pathological", but nevertheless does not minimise the difficulties observed.

The psychopathological point of view tends to emphasise the concept of rupture: in situations in which the patient's mental functioning appears to represent an obvious rupture with his or her previous ways of functioning, the presence of authentic psychiatric disorders can be considered.

How can we establish a distinction between identification of symptoms, demonstration of true depression, and suggestion of the possibility of depression – in the sense of depressive illness – particularly in a context of chronicity?

From adjustment disorders ... to depression?

The patient's efforts of adjustment are the expression of a psychological process designed to preserve mental and bodily integrity, to recover whatever is reversible and to compensate for whatever is irreversible, but also and most importantly to attenuate the dimension of mental suffering and physical pain. This corresponds to the concept of "coping".

The emotional, cognitive, and behavioural reactions triggered by these efforts of adaptation can be described as "normal", inasmuch as they help to achieve the lowest possible level of distress. However, the failure of these efforts could also lead patients to experience difficulties, or even express disorders, described as "adjustment disorders", considered to be transient, situational, and fluctuating disorders of variable intensity, often described as being moderate. They are nevertheless a source of distress and can have major implications on the patient's family and social life.

The patient is considered to display depressive disorders when the permanent presence of the symptoms lowers the probability of their spontaneous resolution, and seriously interferes with the patient's ability to deal with more concrete problems which he or she must cope with in the context of his or her cancer [2,3].

Diagnosis of depression

The observed prevalence of depressive symptoms varies considerably, ranging from 4.5% (6% according to Derogatis [4]) to 58%, and this reflects the difficulty of defining diagnostic criteria of depression in oncology: the more precise the definition of depression, the lower the observed prevalence rate.

Greater emphasis should always be placed on psychological rather than somatic symptoms [5]: depressed mood, feelings of helplessness and hopelessness, loss of self-esteem, feelings of uselessness and guilt, anhedonia, ideas of "death wish" or even suicide, and, in terms of behaviour, irritability and aggressiveness.

The recommendations proposed by the French medical evaluation agency ANAES [6] for the follow-up of patients with non-metastatic breast cancer, which were designed to identify depressive disorders, advocate the use of a structured interview looking for the nine symptoms corresponding to the DSM-IV definition of Major Depressive Episodes: depressed mood, markedly diminished interest or pleasure, significant weight loss or weight gain, insomnia or hypersomnia, psychomotor agitation or retardation, fatigue or loss of energy, feelings of worthlessness or guilt, diminished ability to think or concentrate, and recurrent thoughts of death or suicidal ideation.

In practice, as evaluation of the depressive dimension is intimately related to the organic context, it is often difficult to differentiate symptoms of depression from those possibly related to the course of the cancer and to adverse effects of treatment. Endicott therefore proposed replacement criteria, replacing somatic items by more specific "psychological" items: items such as "significant weight loss or weight gain", "insomnia or hypersomnia", "fatigue or loss of energy" are replaced by items evaluating social withdrawal, anxious rumination and pessimism, inability to regain courage, etc. Particular attention should be paid to feelings of helplessness and hopelessness, often described in the context of the psychological distress observed in cancer patients.

The clinical approach is essential, and in practice is based on simple questions. There is a risk of failure to recognise the diagnosis in the hospital setting due to the short duration of hospital stay, the patients' reluctance to express their distress, and the health care professionals' fear of hearing the patient express this distress, as the general level of conversation is often deliberately positive and combative.

Screening tools may therefore be necessary. The two tools most widely used in oncology are two self-assessment scales:
- HADS (Hospital Anxiety and Depression Rating Scale), composed of 14 items, designed to detect anxiety and depressive disorders;
- GHQ (General Health Questionnaire) for which an abridged 12-item form is available. These two tools do not comprise somatic items.

Suicide

Cancer patients have a twofold higher relative risk of suicide than that observed in the general population [7]. The following risk factors have been identified: advanced disease and poor prognosis; uncontrolled pain; delirium; depression and especially feelings of hopelessness; psychiatric history (particularly previous suicide attempts); social isolation. Male sex and advanced age also accentuate this risk. Some cancer sites are associated with a higher risk of depression [8] and suicide (pancreas, head and neck, lung).

Depression and pain

The anxiety and depression dimension can only be rigorously evaluated after taking into account the possible presence of pain, especially as cancer patients tend to attribute a pejorative significance to pain. Pain management usually leads to the resolution of depressive symptoms if particular attention is paid to irritability, insomnia, aggressiveness and agitation, and non-compliance with treatment.

Depression and fatigue

Fatigue constitutes an extremely frequent complaint in oncology. Can it constitute a criterion of depression in patients suffering from a somatic disease? Is there a causal relationship between fatigue and depression? To what degree do these disorders influence quality of life? Fatigue and depression do not follow the same clinical course; the cause-and-effect relationship between these two dimensions has not been established; however, both of these disorders influence quality of life.

Depression and end of life

The prevalence of depression in the advanced stages of cancer is high and increases as the general condition of the patient worsens. The diagnosis can be difficult in often complex psycho-organic situations. It is vital to distinguish between symptomatic depression, which is responsive to psychotropic drugs (antidepressants and/or psychostimulants), thus allowing an improvement of the patient's quality of life, and a "request for euthanasia", often expressed by the patient or his or her family.

It is essential to take into account the ethical and medicolegal implications in the light of recent media interest in the problem of "medically-assisted suicide", which cannot be likened to suicidal behaviour subtended by undiagnosed depression.

Depression and organic factors

Depressive symptoms can be related to organic factors: the tumour site (primary or secondary brain tumours, cancer of the pancreas, etc.), hormonal dysfunction (thyroid dysfunction, etc.), metabolic or water and electrolyte disorders, as well as iatrogenic factors: corticosteroids, interferon or interleukin, which are frequently used, but also certain anticancer drugs (vincristine, vinblastine, procarbazine, L-asparaginase, tamoxifen). Identification of the factor responsible for the depressive symptoms may enable it to be corrected or eliminated.

Treatment modalities

The management of depression in cancer patients raises two main questions: institution of psychotropic treatment and/or the justification for psychotherapy.

Psychotropic treatment

Psychopharmacological approaches are designed to resolve practical problems of prescribing modalities [9,10] by avoiding possible drug interactions and potentiations, in order to achieve the best benefit/risk compromise. Anxiolytics and hypnotics are widely used, in over half of the patients, to treat the frequently observed anxiety and sleep disorders. Antidepressants are prescribed when depressive symptoms have been demonstrated; there is currently a preference for more recent molecules (especially SSRIs) that appear to be better tolerated than tricyclic antidepressants. Practice guidelines have been proposed: start treatment at low doses and increase the dosage very gradually in view of the hypothesis of a therapeutic response at doses lower than those traditionally required, as well as increased sensitivity to adverse effects. However, few controlled studies are available, and these empirical prescribing modalities need to be assessed in randomised trials.

Psychostimulants (methylphenidate, dextroamphetamine) appear to provide real benefit in depressed patients suffering from pain and/or in the terminal phase of the disease. Although these molecules are widely used in English-speaking countries, their use is limited in France, where legislation prohibits their marketing due to the fear of secondary addiction.

Although a consensus has been reached that a major depressive episode in a cancer patient justifies treatment with antidepressants, no consensus has been reached concerning the management of adjustment disorders associated with depressive symptoms, giving rise to a more empirical prescription of antidepressants. This raises the question of the misuse of psychotropic drugs: Does a symptomatic approach lead to anxiolytic and hypnotic treatments being overused and, as a corollary, are antidepressants underused due to a defect of diagnostic identification?

Psychotherapeutic treatment

Various types of "psychotherapeutic" approaches have been proposed [11,12].

The psychosocial approach can have various dimensions: health education, information, advice, support, reassurance. Relaxation therapy may be indicated. Such approaches can be applied individually or in groups. They must be adapted to the context of malignant disease and must take somatic aspects into account. They often consist of short-term management, requiring the "therapist" to adopt a more active attitude than in non-cancer settings.

Some of these techniques have the advantage that they can be administered by various categories of health care professionals: psychiatrists and psychologists, but also attending physicians, and any other health care professionals trained in these techniques. The psychosocial approach must take into account the family context, but also the social support, including voluntary or patient associations.

The cognitive-behavioural approach in psychotherapy may represent a solution to the difficulties experienced by some patients to adjust to their disease and its consequences. This approach, characterised by the fact that it requires the person's motivation and cooperation, helps the patient to restore a form of control over his/her body and a feeling of mastery over the disease. Based on short-term treatment, it is designed to control particular symptoms considered to be disabling. In the context of depression, the work consists of what behavioural therapists call cognitive restructuring of "negative" thoughts.

It is very useful to combine various psychological or psychiatric approaches. Although many studies designed to evaluate the efficacy of such approaches have demonstrated improvement of depressive symptoms and quality of life, studies concerning the effects of these treatments on survival remain controversial and must be interpreted with caution.

Conclusion

The objective of psycho-oncology today is to deal with the global aspect of psychological distress and to refine its dimensions. The approach to depression in cancer patients therefore requires the definition of precise diagnostic criteria involving specific management modalities. The diagnostic and therapeutic approaches to often complex comorbid situations must take into account the multifactorial nature of the patient's complaint (depression and pain, depression and fatigue, etc.).

Many questions have yet to be resolved in the field of neuropsychoimmunology, and hypotheses concerning the psychogenesis of cancer must be interpreted very cautiously.

The diagnosis of depression in cancer patients therefore represents a priority for all health care professionals, as the management of depression can lead to a reduction of the patient's emotional distress, better adjustment to the stressful events of cancer and its implications, and improvement of quality of life.

References

1   Holland JC. NCCN practice guidelines for the management of psychological distress. Oncology 1999; 13: 113-33

2   Marx G, Gauvain-Piquard A, Saltel P. Anxiété, dépression, cancer: aspects cliniques. L'Encéphale 1998; hors série 2: 66-71

3   Razavi D, Stiefel F. Common psychiatric disorders in cancer patients. (1) Adjustment disorders and depressive disorders. Support Care Cancer 1994; 2: 223-32

4   Derogatis LR, Morrow GR, Fetting J, et al. The prevalence of psychiatric disorders among cancer patients. JAMA 1983; 249: 537-40

5   Massie MJ, Gagnon P, Holland JC. Depression and suicide in patients with cancer. J Pain Symptom Manage 1994; 9: 325-40

6   ANAES. Service des Recommandations et Références Professionnelles. Diagnostic et prise en charge des difficultés psychologiques. In: Suivi des patientes traitées pour un cancer du sein non métastasé, 1998; 84-161

7   Breitbart W. Psycho-oncology: Depression, anxiety, delirium. Semin Oncol 1994; 21: 754-69

8   McDaniel JS, Musselman DL, Porter MR, et al. Depression in patients with cancer. Diagnosis, biology and treatment. Arch Gen Psychiatry 1995; 52: 89-99

9   Evans DL, Staab J, Ward H, et al. Depression in the medically ill: management considerations. Depression and Anxiety 1997; 4: 199-208

10 US Department of Health and Human Services. Guidelines: Acute phase management with medication, 1993. Depression in primary care (vol 2): treatment of major depression

11 Fawzy FI, Fawzy NW, Arndt LA, et al Critical review of psychosocial interventions in cancer care. Arch Gen Psychiatry 1995; 52: 100-13

12 Sellick SM, Crooks DL. Depression and cancer: an appraisal of the literature for prevalence, detection, and practice guideline development for psychological interventions. Psycho-oncology 1999; 8: 315-33

ESO Scientific Updates, Vol. 5
Fatigue and Cancer
M. Marty and S. Pecorelli, editors
© 2001 Elsevier Science B.V. All rights reserved

Psychosocial Interventions for Cancer-Related Fatigue from a Nursing Perspective

Agnes Glaus

Zentrum für Tumordiagnostik und Prävention, St. Gallen, Switzerland

Introduction

Very little is known about the effectiveness of psychological interventions for cancer-related fatigue. Knowledge is still scarce regarding the causes and the complexity of the phenomenon itself. This seems to be true for psychosocial interventions as well. It can be argued that social interventions cannot be seen separately from psychological interventions and therefore deal with the same core issues, even though the term social implies that the person is seen in a wider perspective, for example in the context of his family or work environment. Current discussions about the interrelationship between fatigue and depression or the overlap of the two phenomena show that antidepressive therapy could represent one of the major psychological intervention strategies for fatigue [1], an issue which is covered elsewhere in this volume. This chapter deals with the psychosocial issues surrounding fatigue, with a focus on caregivers' attitudes and psychosocial interventions guided by theoretical models of fatigue. The subject is discussed as multidimensional rather than elemental and an interdisciplinary approach is emphasised.

The readiness of caregivers to address and understand fatigue

In the last two decades of the second millennium, symptom priorities in cancer care have changed and this has been interpreted as a consequence of new cancer treatment strategies such as immunotherapy [2] but also as a consequence of advances in symptom control [3]. Key articles summarising the available, updated knowledge about fatigue in patients with cancer have greatly aided its understanding and encouraged research [2,4,5]. Representatives of the nursing profession have been deeply involved in this process [2,4,6-12]. As fatigue is a symp-

Address for correspondence: A. Glaus, Zentrum für Tumordiagnostik und Prävention, Rorschacher Strasse 150, 9006 St. Gallen, Switzerland. Tel.: +41-71-2430043, fax: +41-71-2430044, e-mail: aglaus@sg.zetup.ch

tom with a major impact on everyday living, characterised by physical as well as psychosocial dimensions, it is clearly of interest to the nursing profession. Noteworthily, mainly nurses and women have dealt with fatigue in a scientific context. In this respect fatigue is not a subject where major breakthroughs can be expected and scientists need to be content with small elements of discovery, which, from a feminist point of view, could be associated with specific female properties.

Having an interest in the patient is a major aspect of caring [13]. Experience shows that, due to an increasing number of publications and educational initiatives on fatigue, caregivers have become more aware and have learned to listen specifically to patients' feelings of fatigue. It can be expected that patients talk about their fatigue if they feel that it is of interest to the listeners. The nihilistic attitude of caregivers who believe that fatigue is the cancer patient's destiny and nothing can be done about it might lead patients to think that it is of no interest and therefore boring to physicians and nurses [5]. Encouraging patients to talk about their fatigue could support the coping process through communication. Being perceptive to fatigue means being prepared to effectively communicate with the patient. Remarks like "I feel well, but..." need to be followed up in order to get to the individual experience of fatigue. Understanding fatigue in patients might represent a much deeper psychological process than assessing and evaluating fatigue for therapeutic reasons. Communication in this sense can also prevent the frequently observed mismatch in perception of fatigue between patients, professionals and relatives [14].

Being aware of and understanding fatigue prepares for the next step of proper assessment and diagnosis. A political, professional discussion has taken place recently about whether the diagnosis of fatigue is a medical or a nursing one. However, this interesting discussion is not helpful to patients: for them fatigue represents a major problem and professionals have to find ways to use an interdisciplinary strategy. Recent research has shown that a very simple instrument, such as a linear analogue scale, can show very efficiently how tired patients feel [15]. This could imply that a simple but effective way of assessing fatigue in everyday practice is to ask the patient, "How do you feel?". It can be assumed that perceptive caregivers from different professions will be able to explore the fatigue feelings in this manner because the approach involves primarily interest, hence a caring attitude [13].

Assessing fatigue does not necessarily provide information about the meaning of fatigue, which can be seen as an important factor if psychosocial interventions are addressed. Little is known about the meaning of fatigue in patients with cancer. We know that feelings of fatigue are sometimes experienced prior to the diagnosis of cancer and may represent the only symptom of the disease, a symptom which provokes anxiety. In patients with advanced cancer it has been shown that fatigue is experienced as a sign of progressing disease and that feelings of fatigue are accompanied by feelings of loss, sadness and grief [5]. The expression "I feel dead tired" could be seen as a metaphor of the approaching end, supporting the notion of energy being a general indicator of health.

Theories to guide psychosocial interventions for fatigue in patients with cancer

Without a theoretical explanation of a phenomenon it is difficult to justify interventions to correct it. Five available models are used here to explore guidance for psychosocial interventions.

The Integrated Piper Fatigue Model

The Integrated Piper Fatige Model [2] is a comprehensive assessment tool which includes 13 different causal concepts, three of which can be seen as psychosocial. The model does not weight the causal concepts. It gives limited guidance for psychosocial interventions. The integrated concepts "social patterns", "psychological patterns" and "symptom patterns" could be used to generate microelements of theory and produce focused research questions. Perception and behaviour could be described as predisposing factors and consequences, respectively, and could theoretically give guidance to test related research hypotheses, such as the relationship between perception of fatigue and consequences of fatigue. This might lead to the development of psychosocial strategies regarding perception, for example on how to elevate the fatigue threshold. Yet, lack of knowledge limits this type of intervention.

The Energy Analysis Model

The Energy Analysis Model by Irvine and Vincent [8] includes energy as a variable with respect to transformation, expenditure, source and energy response modifiers, such as mood and symptoms. All these influences could potentially include a psychosocial aspect and the mood and symptom issues in particular could be used to generate psychosocial intervention strategies. However, the lack of clarity regarding the actions of the response modifiers makes it difficult to work out such strategies. Even though this model clarifies the concept of energy in cancer patients, the meaning of energy remains unclear. The expression of cancer patients "I have no energy" [5] clearly presents a key factor in the fatigue concept and is integrated in many fatigue measurement tools. We have to admit, however, that it remains unclear whether energy, as referred to by cancer patients, has a physical, affective, mental or spiritual source. Nor is it known whether it might be generated by biochemical or immunological processes or by a combination of different factors. This model leaves numerous questions to be tackled by interventional research and raises many other psychosocial energy issues.

The Psychobiological Entropy Model

The Psychobiological Entropy Model by Winningham [4] deals with the functional status of cancer patients, which is supposed to be influenced by primary symptoms, causing an imbalance between activity and rest. At a first level, the model guides interventions in the sense of achieving control over primary symptoms. This is in accordance with other research, where it has been shown that patients with less nausea/emesis experienced less fatigue [16]. In this model the primary symptoms are described as the cause of inactivity, resulting in a rest/activity imbalance and possibly causing secondary fatigue. Secondary fatigue is responsible for a decreased functional status and eventually disability. This theory guides psychosocial interventions directed at such symptoms as anxiety, depression and social isolation. It remains to be clarified whether these symptoms, even if they can be controlled, are not overruled by other, possibly more physical or biomedically-induced symptoms. The model poses important questions regarding the prevention of inactivity, where psychosocial and physical as well as biomedical influences must be strongly interwoven. This is of major importance if a vicious circle is to be interrupted. Whether this can be done, with which type of patients and what type of interventions are effective are matters that need to be further evaluated. The model generates questions in regard to nursing interventions concerning ordinary, everyday activities, where fatigue has a major impact.

The Attentional Fatigue Model

The Attentional Fatigue Model by Cimprich [6] explains fatigue in patients with cancer with increased requirements and demands over long periods of time. Demands for information, treatment impact, coping, changes and all types of worries may exceed the individual's available capacity and result in mental fatigue. The demands lead to focused, selected, and sometimes also involuntary attention to the exclusion of other activities. The consequences are described as affecting memory, concentration, mood and social behaviour [6,17]. This model is supported by work by Grandjean who suggested that structures in the midbrain might present an active inhibitory system; the cortical activity might be reduced by increased activity of the inhibitory system. The reticular activating system (RAS) in the midline of the brain stem is known for its function in maintaining wakefulness. If it is inhibited, the organism is in a state of fatigue; if the activating system prevails, it is ready to increase performance [18].

This model guides psychosocial interventions towards attention-restoring therapies. The aim is to interrupt the continuous draining of energy by bringing temporary relief to the patient's worries and concerns. Properties of attention-restoring activities can encompass fascination, a sense of being away from general things, reducing boredom by extending the scope of current life and compatibility with circumstances/situations/persons [17]. Attention-restoring activities are strongly linked to nature, as nature is seen as a restorative environment. In connection to nature the following activities have been proposed: walking in forests or fields, watching nature – for example bird watching for immobile persons –, feeling the wind, seeing the blue sky, admiring the beauty of a landscape, observing the green colours, enjoying a specific smell, and others.

Furthermore, distraction and relaxation have been proposed to interrupt attentional fatigue. Distraction is considered to be an activity which is different from attention-restoring activities. For example, watching television can distract from involuntarily-directed attention but it may also represent a further "bombardment of stimuli". White noise as a continuous companion may represent further stress.

The model of attentional fatigue guides psychosocial interventions towards the following strategies and aims. Voluntarily clearing the head means deciding to interrupt continuous draining induced by existing problems. The person learns to restore focused attention and thereby acquires the ability to direct attention voluntarily. This should not be done by repressing concerns but rather by facing them and dealing with them. Reflections on life, setting priorities and identification of values may be part of this strategy [6,17].

Causes of attentional fatigue have also been related to symptoms and treatments, especially immunotherapy and chemotherapy, radiotherapy, chronic pain and brain tumours [2]. The model therefore also guides interventions in the sense of symptom control and prevention of side effects of treatment.

The three-dimensional concept of fatigue

The theory of fatigue as a three-dimensional concept [5] can be used as a guide in exploring interventional strategies. In the qualitative analysis of this concept, the physical, affective and cognitive dimensions were identified and the physical ones appeared to be the most dominant in cancer patients as opposed to healthy persons. The concept was developed as a theoretical framework, describing expression, measurement and treatment of fatigue at the identified levels.

Physical fatigue

The identified elements of *physical fatigue* in this concept analysis [5] are converted into goals to be achieved through specific interventions: overcoming or even preventing a decrease in physical performance; overcoming or preventing weakness and loss of strength; dealing with an unusual need for sleep; dealing with unusual, extreme fatigue (as opposed to normal fatigue); dealing with an unusual need for rest. These strategies show similarities with the ones proposed by Winningham et al. [4], with the rest/activity imbalance being a major issue. The hypothesis of a vicious circle phenomenon was put forward [9]. This vicious circle includes unusual tiredness which leads to increased need for rest, sleepiness, activity intolerance, becoming slower, weakness, and decreased physical performance, which in the end leads again to unusual tiredness or fatigue (Fig. 1). Interrupting this vicious circle would be the major aim of physical and psychosocial interventions and this has to be further explored scientifically.

The role of exercise in preventing fatigue in patients undergoing chemotherapy or radiation therapy has been investigated by several researchers and

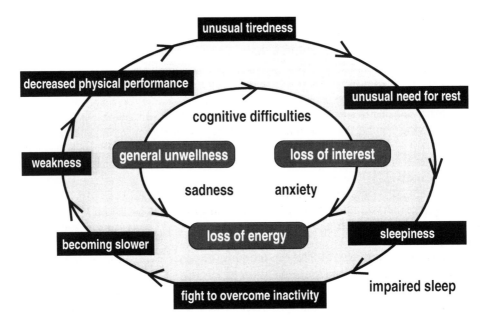

Fig. 1.   Fatigue in cancer: A three-dimensional vicious circle phenomenon?

seems to be promising, at least for certain groups of patients [11]. Exercise as an intervention strategy is discussed by V. Mock elsewhere in this volume. Physical exercise has much to do with everyday nursing care and nurses are often challenged to find out how activating their interventions should be in order to prevent a vicious circle. Nurses know that gentle mobilisation or movement in the bed are most important to prevent secondary disease and also secondary fatigue. However, from clinical experience it is well known that patients often wish to stay in bed, feel too tired to get up or do not want to be activated. These patients sometimes feel totally exhausted after having left the bed for a short period and here the question arises whether activation can still be seen as a type of prevention of secondary disease, maintaining comfort, or whether such activities become a torture. In patients with advanced cancer and large tumour bulk it has even been suggested that exercise might increase fatigue, as physical activity in the advanced cancer patient might lead to an increase in fatigue-inducing cytokines [7]. The interventional strategy could therefore be called "negotiate the radius of action" and this seems to be a highly professional approach which involves body, affect and mind as well as the patient's direct environment, especially relatives and friends. Individual nursing care has to deal with the individual capacity and wishes of the patient and the only solution seems to be negotiation between the two parties after information has been obtained about the impact of activity and inactivity. This represents a psychosocial intervention in itself.

A further strategy addresses the saving of energy or generating energy in everyday care. The highest increase in energy consumption occurs when a patient has to climb the stairs or take a shower [19]. Other activities are less energy consuming and at the same time please patients and therefore generate energy in a different way. For example, when a severely ill person is lifted into a wheelchair and taken to a nice place to feel the sun and the wind and see the blue sky, this is not energy consuming but generates a lot of energy at the psychological level. Nurses and patients should give priority to activities from this point of view and decide together on how they wish to manage the energy account. Creativity has no limits for low energy consuming activities at the psychosocial level of nursing.

The type of exercise may also be adapted to patients with advanced cancer. Headley proposed that seated exercise in a fatigued population may be another way to provide comfort [20]. The author observed that cancer patients sometimes like to experience passive movement, especially if they are immobile. This type of exercise can be seen as physical therapy. Breathing exercises could be part of it and are beneficial not only due to the movement itself but also to better oxygenation of the blood. However, further research is needed to verify the effectiveness of exercise and the improvement of psychosocial and physical well-being.

For some patients, especially those with advanced disease, sleeping, resting and napping seem to be the only weapons against fatigue. In this situation such strategies might need to be converted from weapons into accepted interventions which may be the expression of coming to terms with destiny. It can be hypothesised that coping with the disease also allows to cope with fatigue, and hence to accept fatigue. Experience shows that patients often need to hear that it is allowed to feel tired, and resting or napping should not make them feel guilty. Feeling fatigue has been described by Swiss patients with the word "lazy" and this supports the idea that there is an element of guilt associated with letting fatigue be or become part of life [5].

Affective fatigue

The identified elements of *affective fatigue* in the concept analysis mentioned above [5] are converted into six specific strategies: prevent loss of motivation; reduce activity intolerance; supplement energy deficiency (as described by patients); cope with sadness; cope with anxiety; keep up a fighting spirit.

It has been shown that physical exercise improves psychological well-being and reduces emotional distress [11]. The interrelationship between physical and affective fatigue should therefore not be underestimated. The awareness that they are still able to exercise and the relationship with other patients in an exercise group may in fact represent a psychosocial intervention for cancer patients. The other positive effect is that patients actively use an instrument to confront and combat fatigue.

Many different psychological interventions for fatigue have been proposed. Forester et al. advocated weekly individual support sessions for patients undergoing radiotherapy and reported significantly reduced emotional and physical symptoms as well as feelings of fatigue [21]. Trijsburg et al. [22] reviewed 22 studies dealing with effectiveness of psychological treatment for patients with cancer. They concluded that tailored counselling, providing support according to patients' needs, was effective in the reduction of fatigue and distress and in the enhancement of self-concept. Evaluating the effectiveness of group psychiatric support for cancer patients has shown such support to significantly reduce depression and fatigue and generate greater vigour (in comparison to a control group) [23].

The distinction between fatigue and depression seems of crucial importance in this population because treatment of depression is possible. Overlapping symptoms of fatigue and depression can make this difficult. Visser and Smets [24] have shown, however, that the more physical type of fatigue could induce depression. The issue of depression is discussed by S. Dolbeault in this volume.

Recent research suggests that religious beliefs and similar modifying variables may have a direct influence on the coping process [25]. The sense of coherence as described by Antonovsky [26] may represent a protective factor. Wettergren et al. [27] studied the relationship between fatigue levels in patients submitted to bone marrow transplantation and their sense of coherence and concluded that a stronger sense of coherence was correlated with lower fatigue levels in this population. These new results point to the close relationship between ways of coping and personality traits and the experience of fatigue. This would support suggestions by Weis [28], who designates fatigue in patients with cancer as a sign of maladaptation. The author of the present chapter hypothesises that the term fatigue might present an instrument for repression. It was observed at an international fatigue conference in 1999 that German speaking cancer patients refer to "their disease fatigue", even though the word fatigue does not exist in the German vocabulary of lay persons. It could be hypothesised that it is easier to speak about fatigue than to speak about cancer and that this new term offers an opportunity for repression.

Relaxation and imagery are used to treat various symptoms and side effects. In muscle relaxation techniques various muscle groups are isolated and the focus is on feelings of tension and relaxation. Along with such techniques, focused breathing may be used [29]. Autogenic training has been used for many years to induce muscle relaxation followed by feelings of warmth to promote vasodilation [29]. Imagery uses and depends on mental processes that may enhance relaxation or other physiological responses. All these techniques have been said to reduce side effects of cancer treatment and enhance well-being. However, the effectiveness of reducing cancer-related fatigue by these methods has to be substantiated by research.

Watson suggested that psychological interventions in patients with cancer should represent a selected service aimed at those at risk of psychological morbidity [30]. Some interventions may not be practical or suitable for all. The role of psychosocial interventions in preventing, reducing or learning to accept fatigue has to be further defined. Weis [28] suggests that interventions for fatigue in cancer patients at the level of rehabilitation should include emotional stabilisation through relaxation, neuropsychological training, psychoeducational programmes, and physical training. These different views reflect the fact that psychosocial fatigue interventions are far from being scientifically substantiated but at the same time new options are being investigated.

Since social interventions for fatigue cannot be seen separately from psychological ones, some aspects are to be considered under the heading of the affective or emotional fatigue concept. "Social isolation" has been described as a factor in Winningham's theory [4] and Piper [2] included the term "social pattern" as a fatigue-influencing variable. Social isolation, possibly as a consequence of cancer, could be associated with attentional fatigue, as the scope of a person may be reduced and lead to involuntarily selected attention. Cancer myths still prevail in our society and this may be a substantial cause of social isolation within and outside the family system. Speaking about social relationships and the impact of cancer on them can be seen as a social intervention.

Isolation may progress if fatigue has an impact on the ability to work and the professional role of a person. Inability to work is usually related to the course of the disease and the type and intensity of treatment. It is difficult to estimate the impact of fatigue alone on this. Due to the potential social isolation, giving up working seems to be a double-edged sword. Financial burdens, however, may play a vital role in this regard. In many Western countries the ability to work may be negotiated between patient and physician and financial loss may be compensated by social insurance. However, many patients all over the world have no chance of obtaining financial compensation if they feel too tired to work, for example during the treatment period, and they are at risk of losing their job. If a cancer patient is a breadwinner and there is no security plan for ill persons, giving up work seems to be impossible; this was described impressively by Chan in a Hong Kong Chinese cancer patient population [31]. Social interventions here refer to the activities of assessing the energy left for the professional role and its demands and of counselling patients and families regarding the financial impact of decisions as well as the possibilities and limits of financial compensation. Job modifications may be helpful and a realistic option to explore. A classification of psychosocial interventions in patients with cancer is summarised in Table 1.

Cognitive fatigue

The identified elements of *cognitive fatigue* in the above-mentioned concept analysis [5] are converted into four interventional strategies: preventing lack of concentration; improving clear thinking; improving memory; ensuring good sleep. These strategies can all be linked to the attention-restoring activities described earlier and possibly also to the fatigue-reducing exercise strategies, as well as to all psychosocial interventions described above.

Table 1. Classification of psychosocial interventions in patients with cancer

Individual, tailored counselling, according to needs
Group psychiatric support
Distinction of fatigue from depression
Religious support
Support of coping with disease, foster sense of coherence
Attention-restoring activities; relaxation, distraction, emotional stabilisation
Support adaptation to demands in the professional role, address financial impact
Reduce emotional distress through exercise

Educational strategies to fight cancer-related fatigue – the power of knowledge

Educational strategies can be seen as psychosocial interventions. However, few experimental studies provide empirical evidence for the effectiveness of educational programmes. Nevertheless, it has been generally shown that information and education have an impact on patients' quality of life in the sense of gaining control over the situation and reducing anxiety [32]. This can be applied to fatigue as well. Patients who are informed about the fact that fatigue can be a normal symptom of the disease or a usual side effect of treatment may feel less anxious about it because there is an explanation, which in turn might reduce harmful fantasies. Clinical experience shows that patients feel relieved once they know that fatigue is a common phenomenon in their situation. Relatives who know that fatigue is a side effect or a symptom may be more supportive to the patient. Anecdotal evidence suggests that relatives sometimes misinterpret fatigue, either by expecting the patient to be more active than he or she is or by inhibiting his or her wish to be active. Information might help them understand, and readjust their support.

Education might help the parties concerned to anticipate fatigue and to use coping strategies. In the treatment phase this may lead to preparation of an adapted working schedule, to organising support in the family for specific periods, or to allowing for days with lower energy levels during a chemotherapy cycle. Education may involve instruction about when fatigue is to be expected and what type of interventions could be helpful in a given situation. Specific patterns in relation to chemotherapy or radiotherapy have been described, allowing caregivers to inform the patient and his/her family about the expected impact of fatigue over a specific period of time [33,34].

Counselling involves more than providing information. If fatigue cannot be prevented, living with the restricted energy account becomes an important issue. Stepwise adaptation to limits and possibilities requires gentle and skilful care. When fatigue eventually turns into invalidity, as described in the model of Winningham [4], the energy supply must be provided by others in order to render the quality of the patient's remaining life acceptable.

Table 2. Classification of fatigue interventions in patients with cancer

---

Readiness of caregivers to become aware of fatigue
Information and education
Psychosocial techniques and methods
Attention-restoring activities
Exercise; selected and adapted to specific patient groups
Medical, pharmacological, nutritional and other interventions
Learning to live with a restricted energy account, energy saving
Maintaining an individual activity/rest balance
Learning to accept fatigue within the life context

Conclusions

Psychosocial interventions for fatigue in patients with cancer require an interdisciplinary approach (Table 1). Physical, affective and cognitive strategies are inextricably linked. The existing literature regarding the phenomenon of fatigue has been growing considerably but a wide range of interventions still lack scientific evidence. Considering the available theoretical frameworks, a classification of interventions with eight major strategies is suggested (Table 2): readiness of caregivers to become aware of fatigue; information and education; psychosocial methods or techniques; attention-restoring activities; exercise; learning to live with a restricted energy account and to maintain an individual activity/rest balance; medical, pharmacological, nutritional and other interventions; learning to accept fatigue. Realistic expectations are based on the distinction between the goal of fatigue prevention and the goal of learning to live with fatigue or to adapt to new goals. It can be concluded that interventions dealing with fatigue in patients with cancer require skilful professionals with distinct specialist knowledge and the ability to see patients as individuals in a variety of situations and to meet them as a caring persons.

References

1   Reuter K. Fatigue and depression. Proceedings of the International Symposium on Fatigue and Cancer, Köln, September 1999
2   Piper B, Rieger P. Recent advances in the management of bio-therapy related side effects: Fatigue. Oncol Nurs Forum 1989; 16 (suppl 6): 27-34
3   Donelli S, Walsh D. The symptoms of advanced cancer. Semin Oncol 1995; 22 (suppl 3): 67-72
4   Winningham M, Nail L, Barton Burke M, et al. Fatigue and the cancer experience: The state of the knowledge. Oncol Nurs Forum 1994; 21: 23-36
5   Glaus A. A qualitative study to explore the concept of fatigue/tiredness in cancer patients and in healthy individuals. Support Care Cancer 1996; 4: 82-96
6   Cimprich B. A theoretical perspective on attention and patient education. Adv Nurs Sci 1992; 14: 39-51

7   St. Pierre B, Kaspar C. Fatigue mechanisms in patients with cancer: effects of tumour necrosis factor and exercise on skeletal muscle. Oncol Nurs Forum 1992; 19: 419-25

8   Irvine D, Vincent L, Graydon J. The prevalence and correlates of fatigue in patients receiving treatment with chemotherapy and radiotherapy. Cancer Nurs 1994; 17: 367-78

9   Glaus A. Fatigue in patients with cancer - analysis and assessment. Recent Results in Cancer Research. Heidelberg: Springer Verlag, 1998

10   Woo B, Dipple L. Variations in fatigue scores by treatment methods in women with breast cancer. Ann Meeting Oncol Nurs Society (ONS), Philadelphia 1996; abstr 182

11   Mock V, Hassey K, Candance J. Effects of exercise on fatigue, physical functioning, and emotional distress during radiation therapy for breast cancer. Oncol Nurs Forum 1997; 6: 991-1000

12   Ream E, Richardson A. From theory to practice: designing interventions to reduce fatigue in patients with cancer. Oncol Nurs Forum 2000; 26, 8: 1295-303

13   Gaut D. Development of a theoretically adequate description of caring. Western J Nurs Res 1983; 5: 313-24

14   Tanghe A, Evers G, Paridaens R. Nurses assessment of symptom recurrence and symptom distress in chemotherapy patients. Eur J Oncol Nurs 1998; 2: 14-26

15   Evers G, Nelissen R, Paridaens R. Validity of fatigue measurement in clinical practice. Abstract book 11th International Conference on Cancer Nursing, Oslo, 2000: p 56

16   Pater J, Zee B, Palmer M, et al. Fatigue in patients with cancer: results of the National Cancer Institute of Canada Clinical Trials Group studies employing the EORTC QLQ-C30. Support Care Cancer 1997; 5: 410-3

17   Cimprich B. Development of an intervention to restore attention in cancer patients. Cancer Nurs 1993; 16: 83-92

18   Grandjean E. Fatigue: Its physiological and psychological significance. Ergonomics 1968; 11: 427-36

19   Exerpta Medica. Action on fatigue – A European education and research initiative for oncology nurses. Amsterdam: Excerpta Medica, 1996

20   Headley J, Ownby K, John L. Effect of seated exercise on fatigue in patients with breast cancer. Proc Oncology Nursing Conference, San Antonio 2000, abstr 127

21   Forester B, Kornfield D, Fleiss J. Psychotherapy during radiation: effects on emotional and physical distress. Am J Psychiatry 1985; 142: 22-7

22   Trijsburg R, van Kinppenberg F, Rijpma S. Effects of psychological treatment on cancer patients: a critical review. Psychosomatic Med 1992; 54: 489-51

23   Fawzy F, Cousin N, Fawzy N. A structured psychiatric intervention for cancer patients. I. Changes over time in methods of coping and affective disturbance. Arch Gen Psychiatry 1990; 47: 720-5

24   Visser MR, Smets E. Fatigue, depression and quality of life in cancer patients: how are they related? Support Care Cancer 1998; 6: 101-8

25   Folkman S. Positive psychological states and coping with severe stress. Soc Sci Med 1997; 45: 1207-21

26   Antonovsky A. Unravelling the mistery of health. San Francisco: Jossey-Bass, 1987

27   Wettergren L, Langius A, Björkolm M. Physical and psychosocial functioning in patients undergoing autologous bone marrow transplantation – a prospective study. Bone Marrow Transplant 1997; 20: 497-502

28   Weis J, Batsch H. Fatigue bei Tumorpatienten – eine neue Herausforderung für Therapie und Rehabilitation. Basel: Karger Verlag 2000; 108-20

29   Van Fleet S. Relaxation and imagery for symptom management: improving patient assessment and individualizing treatment. Oncol Nurs Forum 2000; 27: 501-10

30   Watson M. Psychosocial interventions with cancer patients: a review. Psychological Med 1993; 13: 839-46

31   Chan C, Molassiotis A. The impact of fatigue on Chinese cancer patients in Hong Kong. Support Care Cancer 2000: in press

32 Grahn G. Learning to cope – an intervention in cancer care. Support Care Cancer 1993; 1: 266-71
33 Glaus A. Fatigue in patients with cancer. In: Klastersky J, Schimpff S, Senn HJ, eds. Textbook Supportive Care in Cancer, 2nd edition. New York: M. Dekker 1999
34 Richardson A, Ream E. Fatigue in patients receiving chemotherapy for advanced cancer. Int J Palliat Nurs 1996; 2: 199-204

ESO Scientific Updates, Vol. 5
Fatigue and Cancer
M. Marty and S. Pecorelli, editors
© 2001 Elsevier Science B.V. All rights reserved

Exercise Interventions for Cancer-Related Fatigue: Evidence-Based Practice

Victoria Mock

Associate Professor, Johns Hopkins University, Baltimore, USA

Introduction

Fatigue is the most common unmanaged symptom of cancer patients receiving active treatment and also of cancer survivors [1]. The problem of unmanaged fatigue, which affects 70% to 100% of cancer patients, is particularly acute in patients who receive multimodal treatments of high-dose chemotherapy in combination with radiation therapy, hormonal therapy, or biotherapy. Both distressing side effects of treatment and physical inactivity secondary to side effects can decrease functional status and affect quality of life [2]. Despite the recognition of cancer-related fatigue as a significant clinical problem over the last decade, few evidence-based interventions are available to manage this distressing symptom [3].

Physical exercise is a therapy that has proven effective in decreasing fatigue and improving tolerance of physical activity in healthy individuals [4] as well as those with chronic disease states [5,6]. The theory that underlies exercise as a treatment for cancer-related fatigue proposes that the combined effects of toxic treatments plus a decreased level of activity during treatment lead to a reduction in the capacity for physical performance. Fatigue is a basic protective mechanism that is precipitated when there is an imbalance between the demand for energy and the body's capacity to provide energy. A reduced functional capacity means that cancer patients must use greater effort and expend more energy to perform usual activities – leading to high levels of fatigue. Exercise training can decrease the loss and even increase functional capacity, which results in reduced effort and decreased fatigue [7].

Although exercise was a novel therapy for cancer patients until recently, evidence is accumulating to support exercise as an effective intervention to manage cancer-related fatigue. The purpose of this chapter is to review published re-

Address for correspondence: V. Mock, P.O. Box 50250, Baltimore, MD 21211-4250, USA.
Fax: +1-410-2350957, e-mail: vmock@son.jhmi.edu

ports of studies of the effects of exercise in mitigating fatigue during and following cancer treatment.

Review of the research

The first team of researchers to report fatigue outcomes of exercise in cancer patients was MacVicar and Winningham in 1986 [8]. This laboratory-based study compared six breast cancer patients receiving chemotherapy who exercised to a control group of four breast cancer patients who did not exercise and a group of six healthy exercising women who were matched by age. The exercising patients and healthy women rode exercise cycle ergometers three times a week for ten weeks at 60-85% of their maximum heart rate. Exercising patients increased their functional capacity on treadmill tests by a mean of 21% while healthy exercising women increased by 17% and patient controls decreased functional capacity by 2%. Both exercising patients and exercising healthy women showed reduced fatigue scores and mood disturbance on the Profile of Mood States questionnaire, while patient controls reported increased fatigue as well as mood disturbance. The study was limited by its small sample size and quasi-experimental design with non-random group assignment of subjects.

This team reported a second study of 45 breast cancer patients receiving adjuvant chemotherapy in which subjects were randomly assigned to either an exercise group that received a ten-week program of exercise on cycle ergometers three times a week, a control group, or a placebo attentional control group that performed stretching exercises in the laboratory three times a week [9]. Results of this laboratory-controlled study revealed that exercise group subjects (n=14) increased their functional capacity by a mean of 40% when compared with the control group or the placebo group. Subjects receiving chemotherapy protocols that included doxorubicin were excluded from the study, and the study methods did not include measures of fatigue or other symptom experience.

Another team of researchers has conducted a series of studies on the effects of exercise in cancer patients undergoing high-dose chemotherapy and autologous peripheral blood stem cell transplantation (PBSCT). In 1997 Dimeo and others [10] studied the effects of aerobic exercise on physical performance and complications in 70 cancer patients undergoing these treatments. Intervention subjects used an exercise cycle with a bed ergometer for 30 minutes daily and the control group received usual care. Group comparisons revealed a significant benefit for the exercise group on outcomes of physical performance, duration of neutropenia and thrombocytopenia, severity of diarrhea and pain, and length of hospital stay. However, fatigue was not an outcome reported in the study. In a second report, Dimeo and others [11] published the results of a six-week treadmill exercise rehabilitation program in a sample of 16 patients who had been discharged following high-dose chemotherapy and autologous PBSCT. Improvements in maximum physical performance and hemoglobin concentration were significantly greater in the training group than the control group. During post-test interviews, 25% of the control group reported fatigue and limitations in daily activities related to low physical performance. While no one in the training group reported fatigue or limited daily activity levels, no instrument was used to measure fatigue in the sample.

In a subsequent study the Dimeo team [12] studied fatigue and psychologic distress in 59 patients receiving high-dose chemotherapy and PBSCT. In an experimental design, subjects were assigned to a control group or to exercise on a bed cycle ergometer for 30 minutes each day while hospitalized. Psychologic status was assessed by the Profile of Mood States and the Symptom Checklist (SCL-90-R). Patients in the exercise group demonstrated a baseline to post-test decrease in psychologic distress and no increase in their fatigue levels while control subjects reported a significant increase in fatigue levels and no improvement in psychologic state.

In 2000 Schwartz [13] reported fatigue outcomes of a home-based eight-week exercise program for 27 breast cancer patients receiving adjuvant chemotherapy. In this single-group pre- to post-test design, subjects engaged in walking or another exercise of their choice three times per week. Only 60% of subjects were able to adhere to the program, defined as improved pre- to post-test performance on a 12-Minute Walk Test. Exercising subjects increased mean functional ability by 10% while non-exercisers decreased by 16%. Exercisers also reported less fatigue and higher quality of life [14].

In 1994 a study by Mock and others [15] investigated the effects of a home-based walking exercise program and a support group on fatigue and symptoms in 18 stage I and II breast cancer patients receiving adjuvant chemotherapy. Women who were randomly assigned to the experimental intervention demonstrated improved performance on the 12-Minute Walk Test and reported lower levels of fatigue and emotional distress than the control group receiving usual care. Because of the combined exercise and support component of the intervention, findings did not indicate whether positive outcomes were related primarily to exercise, support, or to the combination of exercise and support.

A subsequent study by the Mock group in 1997 [16] tested the effects of the walking exercise intervention on fatigue and other symptoms in 46 women receiving outpatient external beam radiation therapy following breast-conserving surgery for stage I and II breast cancer. In this experimental design, women in the exercise group participated in a six-week home-based walking exercise program during the radiation treatment period. Group comparisons by multivariate analysis of covariance – with pre-test scores as covariates – revealed significantly higher scores in the experimental group on physical function and lower scores on symptoms during treatment, particularly fatigue, difficulty sleeping, and anxiety.

A third investigation reported by Mock et al. [17,18] was a pilot study for a multicenter randomized clinical trial of the home-based walking exercise intervention. This study enrolled 50 breast cancer patients during postsurgical radiation therapy (6 weeks) or adjuvant chemotherapy (12-16 weeks) and randomized them to: 1) an exercise group (EX) assigned to walk 20-30 minutes for 5 to 6 days per week; or 2) a control group (UC) receiving usual care and attentional control. Outcomes included physical functioning, fatigue and other symptoms as well as quality of life.

Approximately 70% of the patients randomized to the EX group were able to adhere to the walking program but a diffusion-of-treatment effect occurred when 50% of the UC group exercised regularly during the study. A *compliance cohort model* of data analysis was used to divide the sample into High Walk and Low Walk groups with 90 minutes of exercise per week as the point of division.

Physical functioning as measured by performance on the 12-Minute Walk Test was significantly higher for the High Walk group compared to the Low Walk group. Mean fatigue scores on the Piper Fatigue Scale decreased from baseline for the High Walk group while fatigue scores increased for the Low Walk group, resulting in a significant difference between groups (p<0.01). A similar result was observed on the fatigue subscale of the Profile of Moods States scale (POMS). Emotional distress as measured by the POMS decreased for both groups from baseline to post-test but these changes were very significant in the High Walk group (p<0.01) and not significant in the Low Walk group.

Quality of life scores on the Medical Outcomes Study (SF-36) varied among the subscales for the two groups over the course of cancer treatment. Self-reported physical functioning scores were equivalent at baseline but decreased at post-test by 48% in the Low Walk group while the High Walk group decreased by only 16%. Social functioning increased for the High Walk group and decreased for the Low Walk group (p=0.01). Scores on the General Health subscale showed a similar pattern.

There was a strong positive Pearson's correlation between symptoms of fatigue and emotional distress (r=0.83, p<0.01) in the sample at the end-of-treatment post-test. There were moderate negative correlations between physical functioning and both fatigue (r=-0.65, p<0.05) and emotional distress (r = -0.64, p<0.05).

Knowledge gained from this pilot study was incorporated into the design and methods for a subsequent multicenter randomized clinical trial that is currently in progress. More than 100 sedentary women with breast cancer receiving adjuvant chemotherapy or radiation therapy have been enrolled. An interim analysis was conducted on 85 subjects who have completed the study. Using analysis of covariance with baseline fatigue levels as the covariate, comparison of mean post-test scores on the Piper Fatigue Scale by intention-to-treat revealed a very significant difference between groups (F=-2.38, p=0.01).

Discussion

This review of the research on effects of exercise on cancer-related fatigue included seven studies of patients during their cancer treatment and one study dur-

Table 1. Studies of exercise in cancer patients

Year	Study	Sample	Treatment	Design	Outcome
1986 [8]	MacVicar & Winningham	(n = 16) Breast	CT	Q-Exp	↓ fatigue & mood disturbance ↑ fx capacity
1989 [9]	MacVicar & Winningham	(n = 45) Breast	CT	Exp	↑ fx capacity by 40%
1997 [10]	Dimeo et al.	(n = 70) Mixed	HDC PBSCT	Exp	↑ fx capacity ↓ complications
1997 [11]	Dimeo et al.	(n = 32) Mixed	post PBSCT	Q-Exp	↑ fx capacity ↑ Hb
1999 [12]	Dimeo et al.	(n = 59) Mixed	PBSCT	Exp	↓ fatigue ↓ psychologic distress
2000 [13]	Schwartz	(n = 27) Breast	CT	Pre-Exp	↓ fatigue ↑ QOL ↑ fx capacity
1994 [15]	Mock et al.	(n = 14) Breast	CT	Exp	↓ fatigue ↓ psychologic distress ↑ fx capacity
1997 [16]	Mock et al.	(n = 52) Breast	RT	Exp	↓ fatigue ↓ psychologic distress ↑ fx capacity
2001 [18]	Mock et al.	(n = 50) Breast	RT CT	Exp	↓ fatigue ↓ psychologic distress ↑ fx capacity

CT = Chemotherapy; RT = Radiation therapy; PBSCT = Peripheral blood stem cell transplant; HDC = High-dose chemotherapy; Exp = Experimental; Q-Exp = Quasi-experimental; Pre-Exp = Pre-experimental; Fx = Functional; Hb = Hemoglobin; QOL = Quality of life

ing the post-treatment period. Two additional studies of exercise where fatigue was not an identified outcome were included because results related to functional capacity elucidate possible mechanisms involved in exercise effects on cancer-related fatigue (Table 1). The types of exercise being evaluated were home-based walking programs, exercise cycles in laboratory or hospital, and one study in which subjects selected the type of exercise. The programs varied in length from six weeks during radiation therapy through lengthy adjuvant chemotherapy (4-6 months).

The study findings were consistent and unequivocal. All of the studies demonstrated significantly lower levels of fatigue in individuals who exercised when compared to randomized controls, to subjects who did not exercise, or to baseline scores. This was true regardless of the type of exercise intervention, length of exercise program, type of cancer treatment, or cancer diagnosis. Exercise effect sizes were moderate to large despite limitations in the intervention studies of small sample sizes that ranged from 14 to 70 with approximately half of those in the exercise arm of the study. An additional limitation was the selection of predominantly breast cancer patient samples.

Studies testing exercise interventions to mitigate adverse side effects experienced by cancer survivors after completion of cancer therapy have also shown beneficial outcomes. Outcomes have included decreased fatigue and increased performance, as well as decreased anxiety and depression and improved quality of life. These studies of cancer patients indicate that exercise can be a safe and effective intervention to achieve physical and psychological benefits, including reductions in fatigue, for individuals with selected cancer diagnoses and cancer treatments.

Practice implications include the responsibility to assess levels of activity in cancer patients who report unmanaged fatigue and to give evidence-based recommendations for managing fatigue – including monitored exercise programs, referrals to physical therapy and rehabilitation, and maintenance of prediagnosis levels of physical activity as developed by the National Comprehensive Cancer Network Practice Guidelines Panel in the United States [19].

Implications for future research include the need for additional research at the highest level of evidence: randomized controlled clinical trials of more diverse cancer populations with a variety of types of cancer diagnoses and treatments across the disease trajectory. There is also a need for objective as well as subjective measures of dose of exercise and of outcomes of exercise interventions. Sample sizes should be larger and based on power analyses. Adherence to exercise recommendations is an essential component about which little is known in cancer populations. The most beneficial type and amount of exercise for cancer patients are yet to be determined. Exercise in cancer patients needs further investigation in terms of other outcomes related to fatigue such as sleep disturbance, weight changes, menopausal symptoms, and immune function.

References

1   Winningham M, Nail L, Burke M, et al. Fatigue and the cancer experience: State of the knowledge. Oncol Nurs Forum 1994; 24: 23-36
2   Nail LM, Jones LS. Fatigue as a side effect of cancer treatment: Impact on quality of life. Qual Life 1995; 4: 8-13
3   Ream E, Richardson A. From theory to practice: designing interventions to reduce fatigue in patients with cancer. Oncol Nurs Forum 1999; 26: 1295-303
4   Pollock ML, Gaesser GA, Butcher JD. The recommended quantity and quality of exercise for developing and maintaining cardiorespiratory and muscular fitness, and flexibility in healthy adults. Med Sci Sports Exerc 1998; 30: 975-91
5   Bittner V, Oberman A. Efficacy studies in coronary rehabilitation. Exercise Testing and Cardiac Rehabilitation 1993; 11: 333-47
6   Ries AL, Kaplan RM, Limberg TM, Prewitt LM. Effects of pulmonary rehabilitation on physiologic and psychosocial outcomes in patients with chronic obstructive pulmonary disease. Ann Int Med 1995; 122: 823-32
7   American College of Sports Medicine. ACSM's exercise management for persons with chronic diseases and disabilities. Champaign, IL: Human Kinetics, 1997
8   MacVicar MG, Winningham ML. Promoting the functional capacity of cancer patients. Cancer Bull 1986; 38: 235-9
9   MacVicar MG, Winningham ML, Nickel JL. Effects of aerobic interval training on cancer patients' functional capacity. Nurs Res 1989; 38: 348-51
10 Dimeo F, Fetscher S, Lange W, Mertelsmann R, Keul J. Effects of aerobic exercise on the physical performance and incidence of treatment-related complications after high-dose chemotherapy. Blood 1997; 90: 3390-4
11 Dimeo FC, Tilmann MHM, Bertz H, Kanz L, Mertelsmann R, Keul J. Aerobic exercise in the rehabilitation of cancer patients after high dose chemotherapy and autologous peripheral stem cell transplantation. Cancer 1997; 79: 1717-22
12 Dimeo FC, Stieglitz R-D, Novelli-Fischer U, Fetscher S, Keul J. Effects of physical activity on the fatigue and psychologic status of cancer patients during chemotherapy. Cancer 1999; 85: 2273-7
13 Schwartz AL. Daily fatigue patterns and effect of exercise in women with breast cancer. Cancer Practice 2000; 8: 16-24
14 Schwartz AL. Fatigue mediates the effect of exercise on quality of life. Qual Life Res 1999; 8: 529-38
15 Mock V, Burke MB, Sheehan PK, et al. A nursing rehabilitation program for women with breast cancer receiving adjuvant chemotherapy. Oncol Nurs Forum 1994; 21: 899-908
16 Mock V, Dow KH, Meares C, et al. Effects of exercise on fatigue, physical functioning, and emotional distress during radiation therapy for breast cancer. Oncol Nurs Forum 1997; 24: 991-1000
17 Mock V, Ropka M, Rhodes V, et al. Establishing mechanisms to conduct multisite research – Fatigue in cancer patients: An exercise intervention. Oncol Nurs Forum 1998; 25: 1391-7
18 Mock V, Pickett M, Ropka M, et al. Fatigue, physical functioning, emotional distress, and quality of life outcomes of a walking intervention during breast cancer treatment. Cancer Practice 2001 (in press)
19 Mock V, Piper B, Escalante C, Sabbatini P. National Comprehensive Cancer Network practice guidelines for cancer-related fatigue. Oncology 2000; 14 (11A): 151-61

ESO Scientific Updates, Vol. 5
Fatigue and Cancer
M. Marty and S. Pecorelli, editors

Energy Balance Interventions: Nutrition and Progestins

Betsy Patterson

Oncology Educator and Consultant, Inman, South Carolina, USA

Introduction

This chapter discusses the role nutrition, hydration, and progestins may play in the fatigue experienced by oncology patients. Research in the area of cancer-related fatigue has had little focus on the influence of nutrition, hydration, and supplementation. While the understanding of cachexia and the terminally ill has received attention, other nutritional and metabolic aberrations in the oncology patient have been less examined. Very little information is available on the multiple and complex nutritional biochemical aberrations that occur with malignancy and the associated treatments. The importance of nutritional assessment and the understanding of which patients are at risk are often overlooked in the oncology patient. Frequently the tumor becomes the focus of care and the tumor host – the person – is lost in the complexities of that care. This chapter supports that the nutritional problems in the oncology patient are multifactorial and complex.

Cancer, fatigue and nutrition: What is the connection?

According to scientific research done over the last two decades one third of all US cancer deaths can be attributed to the adult diet [1]. Cancer is largely a preventable illness. Two thirds of cancer deaths in the US can be linked to tobacco use, poor diet, obesity, and lack of exercise, all of which can be modified by action at both individual and societal levels [2]. What we eat makes a big difference in our energy levels, our mood, and our ability to heal and prevent disease. This chapter will focus on the nutritional biochemical and endocrine aspects of the oncology patient.

When a malignancy develops, new and critical aberrations occur in the host with most body systems being affected. Are oncology patients seen as a "tumor"

Address for correspondence: B. Patterson, 300 Jeff Woodfin Road, Inman, SC 29349, USA.
e-mail: fatiguelady@hotmail.com

requiring tumor-specific treatments? Or has the art and science of oncology begun to focus on the patient, remembering that this is a person carrying the tumor? It is the author's opinion that patient-focused care should be the starting point in all treatment plans. While treating the patient with a malignancy, one should attempt to understand and break down the biological and chemical reactions that may occur, including the nutritional consequences. Having a better understanding of the biochemical changes that take place will lead us to the answers for improvement in fatigue, tolerance to treatment, and hopefully improved survival. If 33% of all cancers have a nutritional connection, then can we prevent the return of that cancer or occurrence of new malignancies by nutritional methods? Clearly further investigation is needed. This chapter will discuss some of the nutritional and metabolic aberrations related to fatigue in the oncology patient.

Who are the patients at risk for nutritional difficulties at diagnosis?

Many cancer patients exhibit changes in energy levels and nutritional status. Common nutritional concerns at the time of diagnosis include weight loss, vitamin deficiencies, and mineral deficiencies. Head and neck malignancies are associated with weight loss, fatigue, and decreased ability to eat solid food. Many premenopausal females are at increased risk of iron deficiency, folic acid deficiency, and calorie-reduced dieting related to society pressure on "thinness" [3,4]. Athletes may exhibit extreme endurance and strength but are also at risk of iron deficiency related to loss of iron through perspiration and microscopic bleeding with their training [5]. The trend towards vegetarianism may also lead to a reduction in protein and to iron and B12 deficiency [4]. Any patient that has a malignancy associated with overt or microscopic bleeding is at risk of iron deficiency. Examples include those with bladder, colon, esophageal, or uterine cancer.

The elderly are at risk of numerous nutritional deficits due to malabsorption and lifestyle factors. One third of individuals over age 70 lose entirely or have significantly diminished capacity to secrete stomach acid. The lowered stomach acid effect on absorption of B12, calcium, iron, folic acid, and possibly zinc appears to explain some of the depletion of those micronutrients in that population [4]. Two common medical conditions in the elderly include B12 deficiency and hypothyroidism: both can be readily treated with replacement therapy.

Alcoholics, the homeless, the less educated, and the economically poor also frequently present with multiple deficiencies that may influence tolerance to therapy and ability to recover. However, the complete list of potential nutritional concerns at the time of diagnosis is beyond the scope of this chapter.

It is recommendable to use a nutritional assessment on each and every newly diagnosed patient, and subsequently have a dietitian see difficult cases and those that appear at risk of developing nutritional complications due to the malignancy and treatment [6]. At diagnosis or early in the treatment phase educational materials should be provided on hydration, diet, supplementation, and fatigue interventions for patients.

Cachexia: The underweight/malnourished patient

The anorexia/cachexia syndrome has a complex pathophysiology that correlates with poor outcomes and compromises quality of life (QOL). The aggressive management of impediments to adequate nutritional intake must be undertaken. Gastrointestinal toxicities including malabsorption, maldigestion syndromes, and delayed gastric emptying are common. Fat malabsorption is seen frequently in patients with a normal pancreas. Approximately 25% of patients with gastric resection and reconstruction may suffer from it. Fat malabsorption can also be seen in short bowel syndrome, chronic radiation enteritis, and in patients with chronic GI complaints who have undergone bone marrow transplantation. Mucositis, nausea, vomiting, diarrhea, constipation; sensory changes including olfactory and taste abnormalities; neuropsychiatric conditions such as pain, anxiety, depression, and tumor or treatment-related anorexia are all frequent causes of weight loss [7].

The cachexia syndrome is far more than loss of appetite and weight loss. Clinical manifestations routinely include anorexia, early satiety, marked body compositional changes with weight loss, adipose depletion, muscle atrophy with weakness, fatigue, impaired immune function, decreased motor and mental skills with decline in concentration abilities. One of the many theories for this syndrome includes heightened cytokine activity (tumor necrosis factor, interleukin 1, and interferon) [7]. An increase in resting energy expenditure may contribute to weight loss in cancer patients. This change in energy expenditure may also explain the increased oxidation of fat. Cachexia-inducing human tumors may also play an active role in the process of tissue degeneration. Important abnormalities in carbohydrate, protein, and fat biochemistry have been observed. Insulin resistance, increased glucose synthesis, and decreased glucose tolerance also have been shown [8]. Such changes are associated with fatigue and have potential to decrease performance status.

Pharmacological interventions for cachexia

Multiple pharmaceutical agents have been tried in order to reverse or control the complex and diverse factors involved with cachexia. Appetite stimulants are the most commonly used medication. Categories of appetite stimulants that have been studied in cancer include corticosteroids, progestational agents, and serotonin antagonists. This chapter will only discuss the use of progestational agents in the form of megestrol acetate and medroxyprogesterone acetate. Both agents are synthetic and were initially used to treat hormone-sensitive tumors. Appetite stimulation and weight gain were consistently shown in several studies of patients with breast, endometrial, and prostate malignancies. Many additional studies have been done in relationship to the weight loss associated with cachexia. Most of the studies suggested improvement in appetite, weight gain, and reverse fat wasting. Few of the studies were able to support improvement in anthropometrics or increased performance status. In the study by Simons, Schols, Hoefnagels et al. the authors conclude the medroxyprogesterone acetate was able to stimulate increased food intake and to reverse fat loss; however, they were not able to show preservation of muscle mass [9]. In 1999 nearly one million prescriptions were written for Megace Oral Suspension. This medication is one of the most studied and widely used appetite stimulants. In the article "On Appetite and Its Loss" by Jatoi, Kumar, Sloan et al. 15 published studies were reviewed. While megestrol acetate was consistently shown to improve appetite, only one of these studies reported a significant improvement in global quality of life [10].

If studies are not supporting improved QOL, is the inconvenience and cost to patients and the health care system worth intervening with medroxyprogesterone or megestrol? Perhaps less tangible or difficult to measure benefits are significant enough to warrant treatment, such as the psychosocial aspects of a patient being able to eat food with their family. The weight itself frequently becomes the focus for the patient, family, and physician. Food and the social aspects of having meals have long been a very important component of life. Appetite is important; ask anyone who does not have one, and listen to what they say! Research is badly needed to develop new agents that will not only improve weight loss, but also improve all dimensions of QOL, including fatigue.

Those that wish to obtain more information are referred to the article "Pharmacologic Management of Anorexia/Cachexia" by Ottery, Walsh and Strawford [7]. This article will provide the reader with information on other pharmaceutical agents for cachexia. The article "Nutritional Support of the Cancer Patient: Issues and Dilemmas" by Nitenberg and Raynard [11] will also supply a wealth of current information on the treatment of malnutrition and cancer.

Obesity: The overweight/malnourished patient

This subgroup of patients with nutritional difficulties is rarely addressed and minimal information was available in the current literature. Only recently has this developed as a concern, particularly in the breast cancer population. In the study by Goodwin et al. weight gain was common during the first year after a breast cancer diagnosis. The use of adjuvant chemotherapy and the onset of menopause were shown to be the strongest clinical predictors of this reported weight gain [12].

The improvement in control of nausea and vomiting has significantly reduced the weight loss associated with the treatment of many different malignancies. The explanation does not stop here; the use of specific medications like anti-estrogens, steroids, tricyclic antidepressants, and selective serotonin reuptake inhibitors (SSRIs) are all associated with weight gain in many individuals. In addition, the reduced activity level during treatment, frequently due to fatigue, correlates with increased storage of fat and decrease in the formation of muscle. This change may not correlate with body weight in pounds but will alter the fat/muscle ratio or the body mass index. Body mass index over 30 is suggestive of increased risk of cardiovascular disease and diabetes [4]. Change in hormone status when treatment-induced ovarian or testicular failure occurs can reduce the muscle-to-fat body ratio [13]. The biochemical changes that occur with malignancy and treatment can contribute to significant weight gain during treatment and for years after treatment.

More research is needed to see the true incidence of weight gain associated with hormone-sensitive tumors that require alteration or obliteration of hormone-specific organs (ovaries, testes, prostate, and thyroid). Education and interventions need to be provided proactively to patients to prevent treatment-associated obesity. Overall, our goal is the elimination or control of the malignancy and long-term survival with avoidance of secondary complications including comorbidity due to obesity.

Vitamins and minerals in the reduction of cancer-related fatigue

In 1940 the Food and Nutritional Board of the National Academy of Sciences was set up to advise on nutritional needs when many young Americans entering the armed forces were found to have nutritional deficiencies. This board produced the first Recommended Dietary Allowances (RDAs). This recommended amount was based on deficiencies and not on levels for optimal health. The actual absorbable value of any vitamin is difficult to predict due to multiple variations in the person's ability to absorb and distribute the vitamin in the body. The amount of a vitamin in any one specific food is dependent on many other factors including:
- the type of soil in which the plant grew;
- the rate at which the plant grew;
- the amount of sunlight and moisture available during growth;
- the stage of maturity of the plant when harvested;
- the conditions and duration of storage;
- the conditions of processing and cooking.

Some commercial farmers are left with precious little topsoil for crops, use force feeding and forced light to speed the rate of growth, and pick the produce before maturity. Has this practice decreased the nutritional value of our current food supply? Again, further investigation is warranted. The recommendations in the US continue to encourage the dietary food pyramid when in reality this pyramid will likely be deficient in some vitamins related to current agricultural practices, processing, and preparation of the foods [4].

In the oncology patient vitamin needs may be altered due to the stress of the illness. Vitamin C and the B vitamins are utilized more rapidly when a person is under physical or emotional stress. For survival during stress, the body must have a steady supply of nutrients. The digestion, absorption and utilization of nutrients during stress may decrease [14]. Chemotherapy and radiation may decrease the efficiency of the digestive process, losing nutrients before they are absorbed. If we combine the decrease in absorption, the lowered dietary intake, and lack of energy to shop, prepare and eat foods highest in nutritional value, we begin to see the potential for vitamin deficiencies in oncology patients.

Folic acid

One critically important vitamin for the oncology patient is folic acid. Folic acid deficiency, also known as folate or vitamin B9 deficiency, is common in the population as a whole, but can be even more likely with persons having cancer. Folic acid is the very important vitamin that is currently advertised for pregnant women and is recommended to reduce homocysteine levels in the cardiac patient. Folic acid deficiency has multiple causes:
- Dietary insufficiency - green vegetables are a rich source (asparagus, broccoli, spinach, and lettuce). Folic acid is also found in liver, yeast, kidney, and mushrooms – excessive cooking can destroy a high percentage of the folate in foods. Folic acid deficiency develops rapidly (over a three-month period) in those with gross dietary inadequacy. Dietary deficiency frequently occurs in the elderly who do not eat fresh vegetables, or anyone with alcoholism. Also patients with advanced liver metastases or liver dysfunction may not have the ability for hepatic storage of folic acid. There is strong evidence that vitamin C needs to be present for the proper absorption of folic acid.
- Malabsorption – the proximal jejunum is the principal site of folate absorption. Celiac disease, sprue, small bowel disease, surgical resection, and intestinal lymphomas all may interfere with absorption.
- Excessive use of folate by rapid turnover or loss of cells – examples include: recover period from red cell nadir after chemotherapy, periods of rapid growth (pregnancy, infancy, and adolescence), myeloproliferative disorders, psoriasis, T-cell lymphomas, hemolytic anemia, and some inflammatory disorders. Moderate to severe folic acid deficiency is frequently observed in patients with neoplastic disease, especially metastatic cancer and the leukemias. The overutilization of the vitamin by tumor cells is believed to be the cause [15].
- Drug interference – it is well-known that methotrexate is a powerful inhibitor of dihydrofolate reductase that causes severe loss of folate coenzymes in tissues within hours [15]. Many other medications can also contribute to folic acid deficiency. Oral contraceptives are associated with a decrease in serum and red blood cell folate levels [4]. Anticonvulsants including phenytoin, antimicrobials like trimethoprim and pyrimethamine, and antituberculous drugs including isoniazid may result in reduced folate cofactors [15].

Folic acid deficiency presents with megaloblastic anemia (the red blood cells appear very large on a peripheral smear) or the bone marrow shows a megaloblastic appearance. The other cause of megaloblastic anemia is B12 deficiency (cobalamin). The mean corpuscle volume (MCV) is the average size of the red blood cells. When the MCV is elevated there is a suspicion that a folic acid or B12 deficiency exists. Because a folic acid deficiency can mask a B12 deficiency they both need to be tested to determine the actual cause of the megaloblastic anemia. Both deficiencies can also occur together. Testing requires a B12 level and a serum or red cell folate level (red cell folate is the better measure of tissue folate stores). The practice of obtaining a periperal smear to determine the actual sizes of the cells is critical in the diagnosis of a mixed anemia disorder. This is often not done routinely and cases of folic acid/B12 deficiency result in unnecessary suffering and delay in recovery.

Perhaps most important for the oncology patient is that a deficiency of folic acid impairs both cellular and humoral immunity. Folic acid is essential for nucleic acid and protein synthesis, and a deficiency will impair the ability of immune cells to divide and multiply. Folic acid can promote DNA repair. When there is a deficiency in folic acid, breaks in the DNA are noted. Recent cancer research has focused on folic acid, particularly in colon cancer. (For a more complete understanding of the complexities of the megaloblastic anemias see reference 16.)

As in all types of anemia the oxygen carrying capacity of the blood is lowered. Lowered oxygen levels in the tissue reduce the capacity to expend energy and to remove cellular waste and CO_2. The heart, the lungs, the muscles and the brain are all affected. Recent reports of neuropathy associated with folic acid deficiency can be found in the literature. With the wide use of chemotherapy agents that can cause neuropathy, supplementation of the B complex vitamins may be beneficial. More research is warranted.

Importantly, no known toxicity of folic acid is documented [3]. A one-month supply of oral folic acid at 400 µg typically costs less than five US dollars. Preventing and resolving folic acid and B12 deficiencies may be one of the many pieces of the cancer fatigue puzzle. It is important to note that a patient may have a low level of folic acid or B12 with no evidence of megaloblastic anemia.

Vitamin C

Vitamin C is another important nutritional component of the healing process. Oncology patients frequently have taste and olfactory alterations. Mucositis is common, as well as heartburn, indigestion, nausea and vomiting. All of these factors may predispose the patient to avoid fruits and juice highest in vitamin C. During the neutropenic phase of the treatment schedule patients are often instructed to avoid fresh fruits and vegetables. The epithelial lining of the stomach is easily disturbed by radiation and chemotherapy, reducing the ability to absorb nutrients including vitamin C. Earlier in the chapter the increased need of the body for vitamin C while undergoing both physical and emotional stress was mentioned. Cancer diagnosis and treatment may well be the most stressful event in a person's life. Controversy exists about the use of antioxidants in patients undergoing therapy. Studies suggest that some high-dose antioxidants may alter the treatment by interference in cell kill by the protective qualities of vitamin C. While further research is needed, it is the opinion of the author that supplementation with antioxidants, particularly vitamin C, is important when the treatment phase is complete. It is well documented that vitamin C promotes wound healing, improves immunity, and may reduce infections. It is also important for the absorption of other nutrients in the body including folic acid and iron. Vitamin C is necessary for the synthesis of collagen and is a component of epithelial cells. It is found at high concentrations in leukocytes. As the levels of cellular vitamin C decrease, so does the phagocytic activity of the cell [14].

Minerals: Iron deficiency

Minerals in the body are numerous and provide complex interactions in the absorption of some nutrients from the gastrointestinal tract. Several digestive enzymes are activated by minerals within the GI tract. Sodium facilitates the absorption of carbohydrates, whereas calcium facilitates the absorption of vitamin B12. All the minerals in the human body are critical for optimal health and functioning. It is beyond the scope of this chapter to cover these minerals. However, one mineral specifically does require some comment because of the high incidence of its deficiency and the role it may play in the fatigue experienced by oncology patients.

Iron deficiency is the second most comon cause of anemia after blood loss. Probably 10-30% of the world population is deficient in iron. In Western countries it is the most common nutritional deficiency, affecting mainly women, children, and the poor. Iron deficiency is a common clinical state in which total body iron is diminished. The general symptoms and clinical manifestations can be divided into two categories: those related to anemia and impaired oxygen delivery, and those unrelated to the hemoglobin concentration, which largely reflect decreases in tissue levels of iron-dependent enzymes. When the intracellular iron enzymes are deficient, epithelial changes occur including angular stomatitis and glossitis, esophageal webbing that may lead to dysphagia (Plummer-Vinson syndrome), and atrophic gastritis. Koilonychia, a flattening or concavity of the nails, is seen in severe iron deficiency and returns to normal with iron replacement [4,14,15].

When impaired oxygen delivery and anemia are present, the red cell has a characteristic hypochromic and then microcytic appearance. On a peripheral smear a few target cells may be seen, and poikilocytosis is prominent in severe cases. The MCV, MCHC, and reticulocyte count are low. Platelets may be increased or decreased [14].

In anemic individuals iron deficiency often not only decreases athletic performance but also impairs immune function and leads to other physiologic dysfunction. Iron deficiency is associated with altered metabolic processes including mitochondrial electron transport, neurotransmitter synthesis, and protein synthesis [5]. Considering that the mitochondria are the "powerhouse of the cell", an iron deficiency could directly contribute to fatigue at the cellular level.

Role of hydration in the reduction of cancer-related fatigue

Water is the major essential chemical component of life, accounting for approximately half of the total weight of the adult body. For good health, water must be consumed every day to replace the continuous losses of water in urine, perspiration, exhaled air, and feces. Humans can survive only a few days without receiving water. Water is an important constituent of every cell of the body, acting as the chemical medium or "solvent in which most of the chemistry of life takes place" [4]. When treated for cancer with chemotherapy, radiation, or biological agents, the body's need for water increases. Many of the chemotherapy drugs received must filter out through the kidneys, causing additional work for these organs. As the radiation and chemotherapy are killing cells, these cells must be flushed out of the body via perspiration, feces, and most dramatically by way of the kidneys. With constipation there is an additional need to drink more fluids. Many of the medications received by oncology patients promote constipation (antiemetics, narcotics, and some chemotherapy agents). With diarrhea, the body also needs more fluids to replace the fluids lost though the feces. Again, some of the treatments given to cancer patients induce diarrhea. Diarrhea can be a result of a drug, infection, or radiation to the pelvis or abdomen. Dehydration is simply defined as too little body water and can occur in uncontrolled nausea and vomiting. Dehydration may result in hospitalization, increasing costs and potential for complications.

Proper hydration is cleary an important issue when treating any oncology patient. In the author's opinion, a hydration assessment should be routine in each visit during the treatment phase. In addition, all patients and caregivers should be instructed on the importance of hydration and symptoms to report when oral intake becomes difficult [4].

Conclusion

This chapter cannot deal with all of the issues that are a concern with fatigue, nutrition, and current pharmacologic interventions. Hopefully it will kindle interest to learn more about the metabolic, hormonal, and energy balance disruptions that occur with cancer and its treatment. Current research has only recently begun to address this important link in the patient's quality of life, tolerance to treatment, and duration of survival. One should be prepared to continually keep up on the research and literature as it is presented. The take-home message from this chapter is to always remember that any patient with a malignancy may develop a nutritional or metabolic problem with their disease and/or treatment. Prevention, early assessment, and aggressive interventions are all necessary to promote wellness, optimize recovery time, and increase survivorship.

References

1   Doll R, Peto R. The causes of cancer. Quantitative estimates of avoidable risks of cancer in the United States today. J Natl Cancer Inst 1981; 66: 1191-308
2   Bal DG, Woolam GL, Seffrin JR. Dietary change and cancer prevention. CA Cancer J Clin 1999; 49: 327-30
3   Rosenblatt DS, Whitehead VM. Cobalamin and folate deficiency: acquired and hereditary disorders in children. Semin Hematol 1999; 36: 19-34
4   Guthrie HA, Picciano MF. Human nutrition. Boston, San Francisco, New York: McGraw Hill, 1995
5   Beard J, Tobin B. Iron status and exercise. Am J Clin Nutr 2000; 72 (suppl): 5945-75
6   Tchekmedyian NS. Pharmacoeconomics of nutritional support in cancer. Semin Oncol 1998; 25 (suppl 6): 62-9
7   Ottery FD, Walsh D, Strawford A. Pharmacologic management of anorexia/cachexia. Semin Oncol 1998; 25: 35-44
8   Mantovani G, Maccio A, Lai P, Massa E, Ghiani M, Santona MC. Cytokine activity in cancer-related anorexia/cachexia: role of megestrol acetate and medroxyprogesterone acetate. Semin Hematol 1998; 25 (suppl 6): 45-52
9   Simons JP, Schols A, Hoefnagels J, Westerterp K, Velde G, Wouters E. Effects of medroxyprogesterone acetate on food intake, body composition, and resting energy expenditure in patients with advanced, nonhormone-sensitive cancer. Cancer 1998; 82: 553-9
10   Jatoi A, Kumar S, Sloan J, Nguyen P. On appetite and its loss. J Clin Oncol 2000; 18: 2930-2
11   Nitenberg G, Raynard B. Nutritional support of the cancer patient: Issues and dilemmas. Crit Rev Oncol Hematol 2000; 34: 137-68
12   Goodwin PJ, Ennis M, Pritchard KL, et al. Adjuvant treatment and onset of menopause predicts weight gain after breast cancer diagnosis. J Clin Oncol 1999; 17: 120-9
13   Reichman J. I'm too young to get old. Times Books, Random House, 1997
14   Kline DA. Nutrition and immunity (Part 1). Nutrition Dimension Inc, 1999
15   Beck WS. Hematology, 5th edition. Cambridge, Mass: MIT Press, 1994
16   Wickramasinghe SN. A wide spectrum and unresolved issues of megaloblastic anemia. Semin Hematol 1999; 36: 3-18

ESO Scientific Updates, Vol. 5
Fatigue and Cancer
M. Marty and S. Pecorelli, editors
© 2001 Elsevier Science B.V. All rights reserved

Treatment of Anaemia in Cancer Patients: Transfusion or rHuEPO

Francesco Mercuriali and Giovanni Inghilleri

Immunohaematology and Transfusion Centre, Orthopaedics Institute Gaetano Pini, Milan, Italy

Introduction

Anaemia is a frequent complication of cancer, especially in the advanced stages of the disease. The prevalence of severe anaemia (Hb ≤8g/dl) differs depending on tumour type (from 10-20% in colorectal and breast cancer to 50-60% in haematological malignancies or in ovarian and lung cancer treated with chemotherapy), stage, disease duration, type and duration of chemotherapy or radiotherapy, surgical intervention, and the presence of comorbidities [1]. There are different pathogenetic mechanisms involved which sometimes occur at the same time in the same patient [2]: aberrant ferrokinetics associated with chronic disease, poor nutritional status, bleeding and bone marrow infiltration, and inappropriate production of endogenous erythropoietin (EPO). Chemotherapy, especially when platinum compounds are used, can be a further cause of anaemia.

Based on a classification by cellular parameters, three types of anaemia can be observed in these patients: macrocytic megaloblastic anaemia, microcytic hypochromic anaemia, and normocytic normochromic anaemia. Megaloblastic anaemia is observed in patients with B12 or folic acid deficiencies mainly due to gastrointestinal tumours; these deficiencies are the result of folic acid consumption by the tumour or of the antagonistic activity of cytostatic therapy. Microcytic hypochromic anaemia (which can be a symptom of gastrointestinal tumours especially in elderly patients) is due to a chronic loss of iron resulting in iron deficiency. In many cases anaemia is normochromic and normocytic, especially when it is secondary to bone marrow suppression induced by chemotherapy/radiation or by bone marrow invasion. In this type of anaemia the mean red blood cell (RBC) survival may be decreased due to autoimmune haemolysis, microangiopathic haemolysis or hypersplenism.

Address for correspondence: F. Mercuriali, Servizio di Immunoematologia e Trasfusionale, Istituto Ortopedico Gaetano Pini, Piazza Cardinal Ferrari 1, 20123 Milan, Italy. Tel.: +39-02-58296444, fax: +39-02-58296447, e-mail: mercuriali@g-pini.unimi.it

In many patients, however, no clear aetiology of the anaemia can be identified, and this suggests the diagnosis of anaemia of chronic disease (ACD). This type of anaemia (which is common in several chronic diseases) is generally moderate and evolves slowly, with haemoglobin (Hb) values ranging between 8 and 10 g/dl. However, Hb values lower than 7 g/dl are frequently observed, especially in patients submitted to chemotherapy and/or radiotherapy [3]. ACD is characterised by a moderate decrease in RBC survival, by alterations of iron metabolism, and by a scanty compensatory increase in RBC production as confirmed by a decrease in circulating reticulocytes.

Cancer patients have also been observed to have an inadequate production of endogenous EPO with respect to the severity of their anaemia as shown by the absence of the expected linear correlation between anaemia severity and endogenous EPO production [4]. These findings suggest that a blunted EPO response to anaemia plays an important role in the development and persistence of anaemia in cancer patients.

The most severe anaemia is generally observed in patients undergoing chemotherapy, who are consequently subject to more frequent transfusions. Although chemotherapy is known to inhibit the proliferation of haematopoietic precursors, it is believed that the main cause of anaemia is a further decrease in the production of EPO due to chemotherapy [4,5]. Moreover, in patients treated with cisplatin, the reduced erythropoietin response is also attributable to the nephrotoxicity of this drug [6].

The results of these studies have stimulated the search for a safer and biologically more rational treatment than blood transfusion in this form of anaemia, and recombinant human erythropoietin (rHuEPO) has been proposed and investigated for the treatment of anaemia in these patients [7]. The rationale for the investigation of rHuEPO therapy in cancer patients is that in these patients the inhibition of EPO production is greater than that observed in patients with comparable types and degrees of anaemia, such as subjects with rheumatoid arthritis or HIV infection [8], and that the erythroid progenitors of cancer patients respond to erythropoietin *in vitro* [9]. Finally, studies conducted in anaemic animals with solid tumours [10] or with pharmacologically induced aplasia [11] have shown that rHuEPO can increase erythropoiesis, thereby demonstrating that cancer and chemotherapy do not lessen the efficacy of rHuEPO treatment.

The clinical symptoms of anaemia are due to the hypoxia-related impairment of most organ systems and their severity depends on the degree of anaemia, the speed of onset, the type of malignancy, and cardiovascular and pulmonary function. Cancer patients already compromised by their primary disease may suffer additional problems from anaemia. In these patients low levels of Hb can give rise to exhaustion, physical debilitation, general malaise and depression, symptoms which, in turn, significantly worsen the patient's quality of life (QOL) on physical, socioeconomic and emotional levels. Anaemia can also diminish the efficacy of some anticancer therapies (such as radiotherapy) while chemotherapy or surgical treatment may be less well tolerated, with a consequent impact on prognosis. Moreover, when a cancer patient is a candidate for ablation surgery, low Hb levels increase the likelihood that transfusion will be necessary.

Since it has been clearly demonstrated that correction of anaemia is correlated with a significant improvement of overall quality of life irrespective of the means utilised to correct it (haematinics, blood transfusion or rHuEPO), anaemia should be recognised whenever it occurs, its aetiology should be determined and it should be treated accordingly in all cancer patients. However, the negative impact of anaemia on QOL is often not only underestimated by the attending physicians – partly because it may be difficult to find out whether the symptoms reported by the patient are attributable to anaemia or to the tumour itself – but also poorly managed because the target haematocrit (Hct) to be reached and maintained to ensure an acceptable QOL in the different phases of the disease has never been established. In many cases it may also be difficult to choose the right strategy for the correction of anaemia.

The aim of this chapter is to provide some basic indications to facilitate the choice between different treatments of anaemia in cancer patients and to define the target Hb/Hct values.

Target haemoglobin values in cancer patients

It is generally accepted that:
- RBC transfusion is seldom necessary when the Hct is higher than 30% (Hb >10g/dl);
- most patients need transfusion when the Hct is around 20% (Hb <7g/dl);
- when Hct values range between 21% and 27% the decision to give a transfusion is taken after a thorough clinical evaluation that is not limited to haematological parameters but includes all factors that should be part of a correct clinical judgement, such as duration of the anaemia, the likelihood of sudden or chronic blood loss, the presence of underlying conditions that might worsen the patient's clinical status, the physical activity the patient needs for his lifestyle, and the presence of a symptomatology ascribed to anaemia.

Moreover, some considerations regarding the effects of anaemia are necessary. A reduced RBC concentration with the same blood volume increases the blood fluidity and triggers the first compensatory mechanism, i.e., an increase in cardiac output [14]. This depends on the greater stroke volume resulting from both the increased venous return and easier ventricular emptying due to decreased peripheral resistance. During this stage the heart rate remains constant. The flow increases equally throughout all organs with the exception of the coronary district where the increase is greater not only because of the increased fluidity but also as a result of the active dilatation of the vessels (this, however, implies a reduction of the coronary reserve and this mechanism is therefore not activated in patients with a fixed coronary reserve). It follows that up to a certain haemodilution limit, the total oxygen transportation is not compromised by the reduction of the circulating RBCs as the increase in cardiac output and flow rate makes up for the reduced oxygen content of the blood.

The second compensatory mechanism triggered by anaemia is represented by the greater extraction of oxygen from arterial blood [15]. It is useful to remember, however, that in most patients oxygen extraction and cardiac output with Hct values up to 35% are normal. With values ranging between 30% and 35%, in patients with good cardiopulmonary function there is an optimal compromise between oxygen transportation and blood viscosity. With values below 30% the oxygen reserves are exhausted and an increase in cardiac output is generally observed; for this reason, when the cardiac output cannot be increased the Hct should be maintained above 30%. Values around 25% restrict physical activity and values lower than 25% represent a risk for the patient and often determine the onset of symptoms of acute anaemia. Some authors stress the importance of taking into consideration these physiological principles together with the clinical conditions and age of the patient, since in older patients (>60 years) with Hct values lower than 30% the risk of silent myocardial ischaemia is believed to be higher due to decreased cardiovascular and respiratory compensation [16]. Higher Hct values should also be maintained in patients with heart diseases that hamper cardiac output increase, such as aortic stenosis, congestive heart failure or atrial fibrillation, and in patients with fixed-rate pacemakers. Higher Hct values must be guaranteed also in patients with a medical history of cerebrovascular accidents and in patients taking medication that interferes with adaptive mechanisms (beta blockers). Coronary failure and chronic hypoxia induced by respiratory failure are other conditions in which Hct reduction might induce myocardial ischaemia.

Some indications can be derived from the experience acquired in chronic renal failure patients. In this setting Hb values of 10 g/dl have been adopted as the essential criterion for starting rHuEPO treatment [17] to reach a target Hb value of 11.5-12 g/dl. In fact, in renal patients it has been observed that a Hb level of 10 g/dl is associated with minor or no improvement in QOL [18,19], whereas QOL begins to improve significantly when the Hb rises to more than 11 g/dl [20]. Accordingly, a target Hb value of 11-12 g/dl could be considered adequate also for cancer patients. However, it is necessary that the Hb values required to guarantee an acceptable QOL be personalised for each patient, taking into consideration all the above-mentioned parameters and the amount of energy required by the patient's lifestyle.

Therapeutic approaches to anaemia in cancer patients

The goal of correcting anaemia is to relieve the physical and mental symptoms related to anaemia; consequently, some form of treatment has to be considered when Hb is less than 10 g/dl and when it reaches levels below 8 g/dl treatment is mandatory.

The first step is to investigate the aetiology of the anaemia and to diagnose possible nutritional deficiencies such as iron, folate or vitamin B12 deficiencies. Correction of these factors may result in increased Hb values rendering blood transfusion or rHuEPO treatment unnecessary.

In case of a diagnosis of ACD the only therapeutic options for correcting anaemia are blood transfusions or rHuEPO. The decision to adopt one or the other must be discussed with the patient, taking into consideration the risks and benefits associated with both types of treatment.

Blood transfusion

Traditionally the transfusion of donor blood was the only treatment for chronic anaemia. Blood transfusion allows immediate correction of Hb/Hct values (an average increase of 1 g/dl in circulating Hb for each blood unit transfused). During the last 20 years the use of allogeneic blood transfusion has been carefully scrutinised because of concerns about the safety of blood supply. In fact, despite the adoption of stricter criteria for donor selection and more reliable laboratory assays for donor screening, entirely risk-free transfusion therapy does not yet exist and probably never will [27,81]. Recent studies indicate that the estimated risk per unit transfused is very low and ranges from 1:2,500,000 to 1:200,000 for HIV infection, from 1:147,000 to 1:31,000 for HBV and from 1:288,000 to 1:28,000 for HCV [21,22]. However, other viral infections can be transmitted. Currently, the most common infectious agent transmitted by allogeneic blood transfusion is cytomegalovirus (CMV). CMV transmission does not pose a significant problem among immunocompetent patients, but in neonates or in immunocompromised patients including cancer patients under chemotherapy primary CMV infection or reactivation of the latent virus following administration of blood donated by a CMV-positive donor may be extremely serious or even fatal.

Bacterial contamination of allogeneic blood has been found to be responsible for 4% of the 182 transfusion-correlated deaths reported in the United States to the FDA (Food and Drug Administration) between 1986 and 1991 [23]. This figure, however, is believed to be an underestimation of the actual number, as only 10% of fatal events attributable to bacterial infections are reported to the authorities [24].

Recently the spectre of transmissible spongiform encephalopathy has emerged with the recognition of a new variant form of human Creutzfeldt-Jacob disease. Unfortunately, with this disease, where even the nature of the agent causing it is not fully understood, the potential risk of transmission with blood transfusion is still unknown.

In addition to the infective risk, allogeneic transfusion induces changes in the patient's immune system that might be detrimental for cancer patients in particular. Alloimmunisation, i.e., development of antibodies against antigens associated with transfused blood cells, platelets or plasma proteins, is the most common adverse effect of transfusion. The process of alloimmunisation is clinically silent but may lead to numerous complications affecting future pregnancies and transfusions including a potential for haemolytic disease of the newborn; difficulty finding compatible red cells; febrile transfusion reactions; and refractoriness to platelet transfusion. The risk of alloimmunisation to red cell antigens after transfusions is estimated to be approximately 1% per unit transfused [25]. Alloimmunisation to human leukocyte antigen epitopes on white cells occurs frequently, with a projected incidence rate of approximately 10% per unit transfused; it is evident in 30% to 60% of patients who have had multiple transfusions [26]. The presence of these antibodies is not only responsible for transfusion reactions but it may delay or even preclude the possibility of organ or tissue transplants.

Transfusion-associated graft-versus-host disease is an extremely severe complication, with a mortality rate of approximately 90% [27]. The condition is precipitated by transfusion of immunologically competent lymphocytes to a susceptible recipient, who is usually either immunocompromised or shares a human leukocyte antigen haplotype with the donor, as occurs most frequently when the donor and the recipient are blood relatives [28].

An additional risk to which the transfused patient is exposed is the immunomodulatory effect of allogeneic blood transfusion. In fact, while on the one hand transfusion induces upregulation of the humoral immunity resulting in alloimmunisation, the cellular immunity is downregulated. Evidence of this is a reduction of delayed cutaneous hypersensitivity, suppression of T-cell proliferation with inversion of the helper/suppressor ratio, and diminished natural killer cell activity, as observed both in transfused patients and experimental models [29].

These alterations are assumed to be responsible for the experimental and epidemiological observation that allogeneic transfusion in patients undergoing transplant procedures results in significantly prolonged survival of both the transplanted organ and the patient. While the immunosuppressive effect can be considered beneficial for the transplanted patient, it adversely affects the surgical patient in that it is responsible for a greater incidence of postoperative bacterial infections and for the fast progression or reactivation of viral infections [30,31]. In cancer patients allogeneic transfusion-induced immunomodulation may increase cancer recurrence and the risk of developing metastases, as has been observed in particular in colorectal carcinoma [31,32]. The role of allogeneic transfusion in affecting tumour recurrences and the survival of cancer patients has been debated by the international scientific community for many years. At present there are several studies that have evaluated the relationship between transfusion and incidence of relapse or survival in oncological surgery, but the results are not conclusive. In early retrospective studies [31,33] carried out on colon cancer patients comparable for disease stage, histological characteristics and several other clinical factors, patients that had received allogeneic blood transfusions, in particular those receiving a large number of blood units, were observed to have a less favourable prognosis than patients that had not been transfused. The prognosis was worse in terms of incidence of recurrences, disease-free interval and survival. These observations have been confirmed by subsequent retrospective studies also in patients with kidney, lung, breast, head and neck or prostate tumours. Other retrospective studies, however, have not confirmed the relationship between transfusion and tumour recurrence and also prospective studies have not provided univocal results [34,35].

The dishomogeneous results regarding the association between transfusion and the incidence of recurrence and the risk of infection, in addition to the ambiguous results obtained in experimental models, have led some authors to deny the causal relationship between allogeneic transfusion and postoperative morbidity. These authors hypothesise that the relationship may indicate that transfusion is an indirect marker of other factors causing morbidity such as age, quality of surgical technique, degree and duration of surgical trauma, intraoperative and postoperative blood loss, and the severity of pre- or postoperative anaemia. Although the immunodepressive role of transfusion in affecting cancer outcome is still controversial, it seems reasonable to minimise transfusion therapy in this patient population by adopting all possible alternatives to increase the amount of circulating RBCs.

rHuEPO treatment

All clinical trials performed so far suggest that in anaemic patients with solid tumours or haematological malignancies, whether or not on chemotherapy, erythropoietin administration is safe and effective. Anaemia is improved in a large number of patients (>50%) regardless of tumour type and of the presence or absence of metastatic infiltration of the haematopoietic marrow [36-39]. Moreover, rHuEPO treatment has been shown to result in a significant increase in energy and activity levels, improvement of QOL, and a reduction of the need for transfusion in patients on chemotherapy with or without cisplatin [40]. On the basis of these results rHuEPO has been approved for therapeutic use in cancer-related anaemia.

Recently the efficacy of rHuEPO therapy in correcting anaemia in cancer patients and in ameliorating their QOL has been demonstrated also in the setting of community oncology practice in which most treatment decisions are not dictated by protocols but are made by individual clinicians. The results of these studies are relevant since, in the setting of postrelease use in community practice, new therapies may not always have the same benefits and safety profiles observed in carefully regulated studies. Very interesting results have been obtained in two similar prospective open-label multicentre studies published by Glaspy et al. [12] and Demetri et al. [13] involving a large number of cancer patients undergoing chemotherapy. A total of 4712 patients undergoing chemotherapy for solid tumours or haematological malignancies were enrolled in these studies. Patients were treated in one study with 150 U/kg rHuEPO given subcutaneously three times weekly for four months; the dose was doubled if the response was not satisfactory according to the attending clinician [12]. In the other study [13] patients were treated with 10,000 U three times weekly for four months; the dose was doubled to 20,000 U after four weeks if the Hb increase was less than 1 g/dl. In both studies the mean Hb level increased progressively and significantly over the four months of treatment to reach an average increase of 1.8 g/dl [12] and 2.0 g/dl [13] with respect to the baseline value. The percentage of patients who experienced a >2.0 g/dl increase in Hb level was 53.1% and 61%, respectively. Further relevant data on the haematopoietic response to rHuEPO treatment can be obtained by analysing the two studies in more detail. Contrary to the expectations, in the study by Glapsy et al. there was no correlation between Hb response and baseline EPO levels. However, in this study a statistically significant Hb improvement from baseline to final values was obtained even in patients with EPO levels exceeding this level. The study by Demetri et al. showed that patients responded to rHuEPO equally well across all tumour types and Glaspy et al. did not observe any differences between patients with haematological or non-haematological malignancies.

Important information on which patients are more likely to achieve an optimal response to rHuEPO treatment can be derived from the modality of Hb increase: 75% [12] and 81% [13] of patients who achieved an increase in Hb ≥1 g/dl from baseline to week 4 had at least a 2 g/dl increase by the end of the trial, and this was particularly true in patients who did not require transfusions. As far as transfusion requirement is concerned, it has been documented by both studies that rHuEPO dramatically reduced (50%) the need for transfusion in all treated patients, independent of tumour type.

In both studies rHuEPO treatment resulted in an improvement of the parameters utilised to evaluate QOL. An important finding was that the studies showed that the beneficial effects of rHuEPO therapy on QOL were mediated by changes in the Hb level. Demetri et al. demonstrated that improvements in QOL occurred in patients who had an increase in Hb regardless of disease response to anticancer therapy. Finally, in patients requiring transfusion the QOL parameters were significantly poorer compared to those who were not transfused during therapy. However, a statistically significant increase in QOL was observed also in transfused patients and the score increase correlated with the increase in mean Hb concentration obtained with transfusion.

The most important conclusion that can be drawn from the analysis of the results obtained in these studies and in a similar study performed on dialysis patients [20] is that the improvement of QOL, regardless of tumour type, disease stage, and intensity of chemotherapy, may be attributable to the increase in Hb levels.

rHuEPO treatment is practically risk-free and convenient for the patient. The same results can be achieved as with blood transfusion, albeit in a longer period of time. rHuEPO is safer than the transfusion of allogeneic blood and is suitable for properly selected patients; besides prevention of transmission of blood-borne infectious diseases, it also avoids noninfective problems induced by allogeneic blood that may cause substantial morbidity, although rarely death.

However, its beneficial effect is much slower than that of transfusion as it takes several weeks to significantly increase the Hb values and more than one month to decrease the transfusion requirement. Moreover, not all patients respond to therapy. For this reason rHuEPO is not recommended when rapid correction of anaemia is required.

In spite of the advantages of rHuEPO in correcting anaemia in cancer patients, this treatment has not yet become common practice and this is mainly due to the absence of guidelines for the optimal use of rHuEPO. Another important issue is the cost of treatment. Guidelines should prescribe the protocols to be used, the factors predicting response to rHuEPO and the selection of patients who could be candidates for this treatment.

Protocol for rHuEPO treatment

There is a general dose-dependent response to rHuEPO, but this response is quite variable in all categories of patients studied. The most widely utilised protocol in cancer patients is 150 U/kg given subcutaneously three times a week. If no response is obtained (defined as an increase in Hct of 6% or more, unrelated to blood transfusion), the dose can be increased to 300 U/kg. If still no response is obtained after two weeks, the patient is considered a non-responder and treatment is discontinued. If the target Hct is reached or exceeded, the rHuEPO dose should be adjusted in order to maintain continued rHuEPO activity. More recent data from the US, using an alternative protocol for a more convenient dosage schedule of 40,000 U SC once a week, with the possibility of increasing the dose to 60,000 U if Hb levels do not rise by >1 g/dl after four weeks of treatment, show similar efficacy and safety profiles for rHuEPO as for the established three times weekly dosage [41].

A number of factors such as infection, inflammation and the tumour itself may result in a suboptimal marrow response to rHuEPO. However, depletion of iron stores is the most important and most common cause of failure of rHuEPO treatment [42]. Iron plays an essential role in erythropoiesis and Hb synthesis; indeed, 150 mg of stored iron is required to increase circulating Hb by 1 g/dl [43]. Thus, it is important to include some form of iron supplementation during treatment with rHuEPO, when the rate of erythropoiesis (and hence iron mobilisation) is accelerated.

The importance of iron supplementation during rHuEPO administration was first demonstrated in patients with chronic renal failure (CRF), in whom a suboptimal response to rHuEPO was associated with insufficient iron availability [44-48]. The results of these studies suggest that the oral administration of iron in patients with CRF is not sufficient to deliver an adequate amount of iron to optimise rHuEPO-stimulated erythropoiesis. Some authors recommend prophylactic oral iron supplementation (ferrous sulphate 325 mg twice daily) in patients showing no evidence of iron overload, and the use of intravenous iron when oral administration is not sufficient to meet the demand of rHuEPO-accelerated erythropoiesis [49]. Accelerated erythropoiesis during treatment with rHuEPO can therefore lead to a "functional" iron deficiency, i.e., the iron reserve may be adequate but cannot be mobilised quickly enough to support the demands of the erythroid marrow. Thus, the quantity of iron absorbed following oral administration may not be sufficient to fulfil the needs of accelerated erythropoiesis, thereby preventing the production of new erythrocytes. The route of iron supplementation and basal iron values are therefore considered to be critical factors in determining the success of rHuEPO treatment [50].

In order to maximise the beneficial effects of rHuEPO it is mandatory to identify those patients who already have an iron deficiency, so that their iron status can be corrected before the start of rHuEPO therapy. In addition, it is important that adequate supplies of iron are provided to support the increased erythropoiesis during treatment. Although some concern exists that certain tumour cells require iron for their growth, iron support should be given at a dose sufficient to maintain all the iron parameters within normal values (hypochromic red blood cells <10%, transferrin saturation >20%) in order to guarantee optimal efficacy of rHuEPO. In our experience [51] with rheumatoid arthritis patients suffering from ACD in whom autologous blood was deposited before major orthopaedic surgery, when at least one of the parameters utilised to evaluate the patient's iron stores was below the 75th percentile of the normal distribution (i.e., serum ferritin <100 ng/ml, serum iron 120 µg/ml, transferrin saturation <20%) we administered 500-1000 mg of elemental iron as iron sucrose before starting rHuEPO treatment. The total cumulative dose was subdivided into four to five daily doses. Moreover, during rHuEPO treatment at each autologous donation 200 mg of elemental iron was administered by slow intravenous infusion.

During rHuEPO treatment it is recommended to monitor the iron status by monthly determination of serum ferritin, serum iron and total iron binding capacity; moreover, when a Coulter counter is available, it would be very useful to check the appearance and the percentage of hypochromic RBCs in the circulation prior to laboratory evidence of depletion of iron stores [48].

The Hb/Hct should be determined every week at the beginning of treatment until the target level is reached, every two weeks until the values are stabilised, and then at monthly intervals.

Factors affecting rHuEPO response in cancer patients

While rHuEPO is effective in correcting anaemia, increasing QOL and reducing transfusion requirement in patients with solid and haematological malignancies, the response rates are variable. This factor, along with the high cost of rHuEPO treatment, calls for accurate selection of patients who are more likely to respond to rHuEPO. For this purpose it is necessary to identify factors that could predict easily and possibly at low cost a favourable response to rHuEPO therapy in cancer patients. Several factors have been investigated including type of chemotherapy, bone marrow involvement, serum EPO levels, reticulocytes, soluble transferrin receptors (TfRs), and iron status.

Chemotherapy and residual marrow function

The effect of the type and intensity of chemotherapy and bone marrow involvement was investigated in two multicentre placebo-controlled trials in anaemic patients (Hct <32%) receiving cisplatin and noncisplatin chemotherapy for the treatment of cancer [36,52]. Differences in the response to rHuEPO could not be attributed to differences in the type or intensity of chemotherapy as evaluated by the degree of neutropenia or thrombocytopenia. In these studies no differences in these parameters were observed between patients who responded to rHuEPO therapy and those who did not, except in myelodysplasia where the response to rHuEPO was very poor. However, a platelet count >150x10^9/L associated with a low baseline EPO level has been reported to be an acceptable predictor of favourable response in anaemic patients with multiple myeloma and non-Hodgkin's lymphoma [53].

Serum EPO levels

Baseline serum EPO levels do not seem to be significant predictors of response to rHuEPO treatment [54,55]. The inappropriateness of absolute values of serum EPO as a predictor of response could be due to the considerable fluctuation in serum EPO levels caused by chemotherapy, to the wide physiological range of serum EPO levels, and to the loss of an inverse correlation between serum EPO and Hb levels due to an inadequate EPO response to the degree of anaemia in cancer patients.

The definition of this inadequate response to the degree of anaemia can be obtained from a comparison between the patient's serum EPO value and the reference serum EPO threshold values for that degree of anaemia [56]. Adequacy of EPO response to anaemia can be evaluated in an individual patient through the observed/predicted (O/P) log (EPO) ratio. The predicted serum EPO value is derived from reference regression at a particular Hct or Hb level [57]. The O/P ratio allows clinicians to determine the inadequacy of the EPO response in individual patients and has the advantage of providing a measure of the magnitude of inadequacy [56].

Indicators of early response

Variations in Hb level after two weeks of rHuEPO treatment proved to be a useful indicator of response in two clinical studies [53,58]. Several factors, however, may affect the Hb levels in cancer patients undergoing chemotherapy, and therefore Hb variations at two weeks are useless as response parameters in individual subjects. In such cases reticulocyte count, red cell indexes, or circulating transferrin receptor [48] might prove useful in establishing criteria for early response.

A soluble form of transferrin receptor is present in human serum [59]. The available evidence indicates that serum transferrin receptor is a truncated form of surface receptor. Its major source is the erythroid precursors in the bone mar-row and an increase in serum level correlates with an increase in bone marrow activity. Thus, the serum transferrin receptor assay, together with the reticulo-cyte count, may be the method of choice for evaluating total erythroid marrow activity in the clinical setting, particularly when serial assessments are needed, such as in monitoring the erythropoietic response to rHuEPO [60].

Algorithms for response prediction

Ludwig et al. [58] found that after two weeks of treatment serum EPO (<100 mU/ml) and change in Hb (≥0.5 g/dl) taken together were a powerful predictor of response to rHuEPO treatment. Cazzola et al. [53] developed a similar algo-rithm for predicting response by using the baseline serum EPO level and O/P ra-tio, taken as indicators of adequacy of endogenous EPO production, and varia-tion in Hb level after two weeks, taken as an early indicator of response. The use of this algorithm in patients treated with 5000 or 10,000 U of rHuEPO has a sensitivity of 88%, a specificity of 93%, and an overall accuracy of 90%. More-over, preliminary data suggest that the use of variation in circulating transfer-rin receptor after two weeks may further improve the predictive power of the above algorithm.

Conclusions

Anaemia is a frequent complication of cancer. Cancer patients already compro-mised by their primary disease may have additional problems due to anaemia. Anaemia should therefore be diagnosed and treated in order to improve the QOL of these patients. The most common form of anaemia that occurs with ma-lignancy is anaemia of chronic disease.

   Traditionally the transfusion of allogeneic blood was the only treatment for chronic anaemia. At present it is possible to obtain the benefit of blood transfu-sion by physiologically stimulating bone marrow function with rHuEPO. It is universally accepted that rHuEPO treatment is a safe and effective means of increasing the circulating RBC mass in patients with various types of anaemia due to absolute and relative EPO deficiency.

   This important physiological effect has been confirmed in more than 60% of cancer patients and has been shown to result in correction of anaemia, improve-ment of QOL and reduction of the need for allogeneic blood transfusions. This is particularly important in cancer patients, in whom transfusion could reduce the immunocompetence and adversely affect disease outcome. However, rHuEPO in the treatment of cancer patients is not being used to its full potential. One of the reasons for this could be the underestimation of the role of anaemia in cancer patients who are either undergoing chemotherapy or are candidates for surgery. Other reasons could be the need for physicians to better understand the role of rHuEPO in correcting anaemia, and to know how they could optimise the use of rHuEPO in order to achieve acceptable Hb values.

Since 30% to 40% of cancer patients do not respond to rHuEPO [13,61], it is important to identify clinical or laboratory parameters that, at an acceptable cost, could identify those patients who are most likely to respond to treatment. Many parameters have been considered and several algorithms to predict response have been developed. Although these treatment algorithms appear to be useful, the prediction of response of the single patient is still very imprecise. It will be necessary to confirm the results obtained in carefully controlled and monitored studies with these algorithms or with the utilisation of other parameters in the setting of community oncology practice.

Another important issue regarding the use of rHuEPO is its cost effectiveness, especially in comparison with the cost effectiveness of blood transfusion. One study demonstrated significantly (p<0.001) greater increases in Hb level in rHuEPO-treated patients (2.2 g/dl) than in placebo-treated patients (0.5 g/dl) receiving nonplatinum chemotherapy, despite a significantly (p=0.0057) higher transfusion rate in the placebo group (39.5%) than in the rHuEPO group (24.7%) [62]. Using Hb level as the measure of effectiveness, Cremieux et al. [63] in 1999 noted that rHuEPO treatment was cost-effective relative to standard care (i.e., blood transfusions). This finding was based on an analysis of published data on 290 patients from a phase III randomised, double-blind, placebo-controlled trial [52,54] and approximately 4500 patients from two separate open-label, non-randomised, community-based trials of rHuEPO [12,13]. Specifically, in the randomised controlled trial the effectiveness achieved with US $ 1 spent on standard care could be achieved with only $ 0.81 of rHuEPO care. Results from the community trials were qualitatively similar, with $ 0.70 to $ 0.78 of rHuEPO therapy yielding $ 1 of standard-care effectiveness. Specific changes in Hb levels reported in the studies were 0.4 g/dl for the placebo-treated patients in the controlled study [52,54] vs 2.1 g/dl for the rHuEPO-treated patients in the same study, 1.8 g/dl for patients in one of the two community studies [12] and 2.0 g/dl for patients in the second community study [13]. These findings suggested that rHuEPO is approximately 20% to 25% more cost-effective than transfusions when the endpoint is the Hb level. A subsequent study by the same investigators suggested further that cost differences between rHuEPO and transfusion might be even greater, as the cost per unit of blood ($ 354) in the original study [63] was 28% below that determined in the more recent study ($ 491) [64]. Obviously, greater cost-effectiveness of rHuEPO, compared with blood transfusions, would be a consideration for physicians deciding on treatment for cancer-related anaemia.

References

1   Van Camp B. Anemia in cancer. Erythropoiesis 1991; 2: 39-40
2   Spivak JL: Cancer related anemia: Its causes and characteristics. Semin Oncol 1994; 21 (suppl 3): 3-8

3   Case DC Jr, Sears DA. Anemia of chronic disease: spectrum of associated diseases in a series of unselected hospitalised patients. Am J Med 1989; 87: 639-46

4   Miller CB, Jones RJ, Piantadosi S, Abeloff MD, Spivak JL. Decreased erythropoietin response in patients with the anemia of cancer. N Engl J Med 1990, 322: 1689-2

5   Birgegard G, Wide L, Simonson B. Marked erythropoietin increase before fall in Hb after treatment with cytostatic drugs suggests mechanism other than anemia for stimulation. Br J Haematol 1989; 72: 564-6

6   Wood P, Nygaand S, Hrushesky WJM. Cisplatin-induced anemia is correctable with erythropoietin. Blood 1988; 72 (suppl): 52

7   Bukowski RM. Clinical efficacy of recombinant human erythropoietin (r-HuEPO) in the treatment of anemia associated with cancer. Erythropoiesis 1994; 5: 108-14

8   Spivak JL. Rationale for the use of recombinant human erythropoietin (r-HuEPO) in the management of anemic cancer patients. Erythropoiesis 1994; 5: 101-7

9   Dainiak N, Kulkarni V, Howard D, Kalmanti M, Dewey MC, Hoffman R. Mechanisms of abnormal erythropoiesis in malignancy. Cancer 1983; 51: 1101

10   DeGowin RL, Gibson DP. Erythropoietin and the anemia of mice bearing extramedullary tumor. J Lab Clin Med 1979; 94: 303

11   Reissman KR, Udupa KB. Effect of erythropoietin on proliferation of erythropoietin-responsive cells. Cell Tissue Kinet 1972; 5: 481-7

12   Glapsy J, Bukowski R, Steinberg D, et al. Impact of therapy with epoetin alfa on clinical outcomes in patients with nonmyeloid malignancies during cancer chemotherapy in community oncology practice. J Clin Oncol 1997; 15: 1218-34

13   Demetri GD, Kris M, Wade J, et al. Quality of life benefit in chemotherapy patients treated with epoetin alfa is independent of disease response or tumor type: results from a prospective community oncology study. J Clin Oncol 1998; 16: 3412-25

14   Tuman KJ. Tissue oxygen delivery: the physiology of anemia. Anaest Clin North Am 1990; 9: 451-69

15   Rodman T, Close HP, Purcell MK. The oxyhemoglobin dissociation curve in anemia. Ann Intern Med 1960; 52: 295-309

16   Welch HG, Meehan KR, Goodnough LT. Prudent strategies for elective red blood cell transfusion. Ann Int Med 1992; 116: 393-402

17   Koene RAP, Frenken LAM. Starting r-HuEPO in chronic renal failure: when, why, and how? Nephrol Dial Transplant 1995;10 (suppl 2): 35-42

18   Levin NW, Lazarus JM, Nissenson AR. National cooperative rHu erythropoietin study in patients with chronic renal failure – an interim report. Am J Kidney Dis 1993; 22 (suppl 1): 3-12

19   Ifudu O, Paul H, Mayers JD, et al. Pervasive failed rehabilitation in center-based maintenance hemodialysis patients. Am J Kidney Dis 1994; 23: 394-400

20   Moreno F, Valderrabano F, Aracil FJ, et al. Influence of haematocrit on quality of life of haemodialysis patients. Abstracts Annual EDTA-ERA Congress, Vienna 1994

21   Lackritz EM, Satten GA, Aberle-Grasse J, et al. Estimated risk of transmission of the human immunodeficiency virus by screened blood in the United States. N Engl J Med 1995; 333: 1721-5

22   Schreiber GB, Busch MP, Kleinman SH, Korelitz JJ. The risk of transfusion-transmitted viral infections. The Retrovirus Epidemiology Donor Study. N Engl J Med 1996; 334: 1685-90

23   Menitove JE. Transfusion-transmitted infections: update. Semin Hematol 1996; 33: 290-301

24   Sazama K. Bacteria in blood for transfusion. Arch Pathol Lab Med 1994; 118: 350-64

25   Heddle NM, Soutar RL, O'Hoski PL, et al. A prospective study to determine the frequency and clinical significance of alloimmunization post-transfusion. Br J Haematol 1995; 91: 1000-5

26   Mollison PL, Engelfriet CP, Contreras M. Blood transfusion in clinical medicine, 9th ed. Oxford: Blackwell Scientific Publications, 1993

27 Anderson KC, Weinstein HJ. Transfusion-associated graft-versus-host disease. N Engl J Med 1990; 323: 315-21

28 Ohto H, Anderson KC. Survey of transfusion-associated graft-versus-host disease in immunocompetent recipients. Transfus Med Rev 1996; 10: 31-43

29 Gascon P, Zoumbos NC, Young NS. Immunological abnormalities in patients receiving multiple blood transfusions. Ann Intern Med 1984; 100: 173-7

30 Blumberg N, Heal JM. Effects of transfusion on immune function. Cancer recurrence and infection. Arch Pathol Lab Med 1994; 118: 371-9

31 Blumberg N. Allogeneic transfusion and infections: economic and clinical implications. Semin Hematol 1997; 34 (suppl 2): 34-40

32 Tartter PI. The association of perioperative blood transfusion with colorectal cancer recurrence. Ann Surg 1992; 216: 633-8

33 Creasy TS, Veitch PS, Bell PR. A relationship between perioperative blood transfusion and recurrence of carcinoma of the sigmoid colon following potentially curative surgery. Ann R Coll Surg Engl 1987; 69: 100-3

34 Heiss MM, Mempel W, Delanoff C, et al. Blood transfusion modulated tumor recurrence: first results of randomized study of autologous versus allogeneic blood transfusion in colorectal cancer surgery. J Clin Oncol 1994; 12: 1859-67

35 Houbiers JG, Brand A, van de Watering LM, et al. Randomized controlled trial comparing transfusion of leucocyte-depleted or buffy-coat depleted blood in surgery for colorectal cancer. Lancet 1994; 344: 573-8

36 Abels RI, Larholt KM, Krantz KD, Bryant EC. Recombinant human erythropoietin (r-HuEPO) for the treatment of the anemia of cancer. In: Murphy MJ Jr, ed. Blood cell growth factors: Their present and future use in hematology and oncology. Proceedings of the Beijing Symposium, Dayton, Ohio: Alpha Med Press, 1991; 121-41

37 Bukowski RM. Clinical efficacy of recombinant human erythropoietin (r-HuEPO) in the treatment of anemia associated with cancer. Erythropoiesis 1994; 5: 108-14

38 Ludwig H, Fritz E, Leitgeb C, et al. Erythropoietin treatment for chronic anemia of selected hematological malignancies and solid tumors. Ann Oncol 1993; 4: 161-7

39 Miller CB, Platanias LC, Mills SR, et al. Phase I-II trial of erythropoietin in the treatment of cisplatin-associated anemia. J Natl Cancer Inst 1992; 84: 98-103

40 Goodnough LT, Anderson KC, Kurtz S, et al. Indications and guidelines for the use of hematopoietic growth factors. Transfus 1993; 33: 944-59

41 Gabrilove JL, Cleeland CS, Livingston RB, Sarokhan B, Winer E, Einhorn LH. Clinical evaluation of once-weekly dosing of epoetin alfa in chemotherapy patients: improvements in hemoglobin and quality of life are similar to three-times-weekly dosing. J Clin Oncol 2001; 19 (in press)

42 Sunder-Plassmann G, Hörl WH. Iron metabolism and iron substitution during erythropoietin therapy. Clin Invest 1994; 72: S111-5

43 Cook JD, Skikne BS, Lynch SR, Reusser ME. Estimates of iron sufficiency in the US population. Blood 1986; 68: 726-31

44 Anastassiades EG, Howarth D, Howarth J, et al. Monitoring of iron requirements in renal patients on erythropoietin. Nephrol Dial Transplant 1993; 8: 846-53

45 Eschbach JW, Kelly MR, Haley NR, et al. Treatment of the anemia of progressive renal failure with recombinant human erythropoietin. N Engl J Med 1989; 321: 158-63

46 Bergamann M, Grütxmacher P, Heuser J, Kalwasser JP. Iron metabolism under rHuEPO therapy in patients on maintenance hemodialysis. Int J Artif Organs 1990; 13: 109-12

47 Brugnara C, Colella GM, Cremins J, et al. Effects of subcutaneous recombinant human erythropoietin in normal subjects: development of decreased reticulocyte hemoglobin content and iron deficient erythropoiesis. J Lab Clin Med 1994; 123: 660-6

48 Brugnara C, Chambers LA, Malynn E, Goldberg MA, Kruskall MS. Red blood cell regeneration induced by subcutaneous recombinant erythropoietin: Iron-deficient erythropoiesis in iron-replete subjects. Blood 1993; 81: 956-64

49 Van Wyck DB. Iron management during recombinant human erythropoietin therapy. Am J Kidney Dis 1989; 14 (suppl 1): 9-13
50 Mercuriali F, Zanella A, Barosi G, et al. Use of erythropoietin to increase the volume of autologous blood donated by orthopedic patients. Transfusion 1993; 33: 55-60
51 Mercuriali F, Gualtieri G, Sinigaglia L, et al. Use of recombinant human erythropoietin to assist autologous blood donation by anemic rheumatoid arthritis patients undergoing major orthopedic surgery. Transfusion 1994; 34: 501-6
52 Abels R. Erythropoietin for anemia in cancer patients. Eur J Cancer 1993; 29A (suppl 2): S2-8
53 Cazzola M, Messinger D, Battistel V, et al. Recombinant human erythropoietin in anemia associated with multiple myeloma or non-Hodgkin lymphoma: dose finding and identification of predictors of response. Blood 1995; 86: 4446-53
54 Case DC Jr, Bukowski RM, Carey RW, et al. Recombinant human erythropoietin therapy for anemic cancer patients on combination chemotherapy. J Natl Cancer Inst 1993; 85: 801-6
55 Platanias LC, Miller CB, Mick C, et al. Treatment of chemotherapy-induced anemia with recombinant human erythropoietin in cancer patients. J Clin Oncol 1991; 9: 2021-6
56 Barosi G, Cazzola M, De Vincentiis A, et al. Guidelines for the use of recombinant human erythropoietin. Haematologica 1994; 79: 526-33
57 Beguin Y, Clemons G, Pootrakul P, Fillet G. Quantitative assessment of erythropoiesis and functional classification of anemia based on measurements of serum transferrin receptor and erythropoietin. Blood 1993; 81: 1067-76
58 Ludwig H, Fritz E, Leitgeb C, et al. Prediction of response to erythropoietin treatment in chronic anemia of cancer. Blood 1994; 84: 1056-63
59 Huebers HA, Beguin Y, Pootrakul P, et al. Intact transferrin receptors in human plasma and their relation to erythropoiesis. Blood 1990; 75: 102-7
60 Cazzola M, Ponchio L, Beguin Y, et al. Subcutaneous erythropoietin for treatment of refractory anemia in hematologic disorders. Results of a phase I/II clinical trial. Blood 1992; 79: 29-37
61 Littlewood TJ, Bajetta E, Nortier JWR, Rapoport B, for the Epoetin Alfa Study Group. Effects of epoetin alfa on hematologic parameters and quality of life in cancer patients receiving nonplatinum chemotherapy: results of a randomized, double-blind, placebo-controlled trial. J Clin Oncol 2001 (in press)
62 Littlewood TJ, Bajetta E, Cella D. Efficacy and quality of life outcomes of epoetin alfa in a double-blind, placebo-controlled multicenter study of cancer patients receiving non-platinum containing chemotherapy. Proc Am Soc Clin Oncol 1999; 18: 574a (abstract)
63 Cremieux P-Y, Finkelstein SN, Berndt ER, et al. Cost effectiveness, quality-adjusted life-years and supportive care. Pharmacoeconomics 1999; 16: 459-72
64 Cremieux P-Y, Barrett B, Anderson K, et al. Cost of outpatient blood transfusion in cancer patients. J Clin Oncol 2000; 18: 2755-61

ESO Scientific Updates, Vol. 5
Fatigue and Cancer
M. Marty and S. Pecorelli, editors
© 2001 Elsevier Science B.V. All rights reserved

Cancer-Related Fatigue: Clinical Screening, Assessment and Management

Lynne Wagner-Raphael and David Cella

Evanston Northwestern Healthcare, Evanston, Illinois, USA, and Robert H. Lurie Comprehensive Cancer Center of Northwestern University, Chicago, Illinois, USA

Introduction

Due to recent medical advances, the life expectancy of people with cancer has been increasing. Given this, treatment interventions that effectively manage cancer-related symptoms and improve the quality of life of cancer survivors are needed. People with cancer experience many symptoms due to their illness and its treatments. Cancer-related fatigue is the most prevalent symptom associated with cancer, resulting in significant morbidity, functional impairments, and reduced quality of life. If fatigue could be effectively managed, the overall symptom burden of cancer would be dramatically reduced.

Diagnostic criteria for cancer-related fatigue

The Fatigue Coalition, a multidisciplinary group of medical practitioners, researchers, and patient advocates, developed a working set of diagnostic criteria for cancer-related fatigue, which was published in 1998 [1]. These criteria are presented in Table 1.

Prevalence of cancer-related fatigue

Cancer-related fatigue is the most prevalent symptom associated with cancer [2-4]. The prevalence of reported fatigue in cancer patients has been estimated to be between 60% and 90% of patients, depending on the patient sample and methodology employed [3,5-10]. Cella (unpublished data) found that 76% of

---

Address for correspondence: L. Wagner-Raphael, Northwestern University, 339 E. Chicago Ave., Office 717, Chicago, IL 60611, USA.
e-mail: l-wagner-raphael@northwestern.edu

Table 1. Proposed ICD-10 criteria for cancer-related fatigue (1998 Draft) [1]

A. Six (or more) of the following symptoms have been present every day or nearly every day during the same 2-week period in the past month, and at least one of the symptoms is (1) significant fatigue.

    1. Significant fatigue, diminished energy, or increased need to rest, disproportionate to any recent change in activity level;
    2. Complaints of generalized weakness or limb heaviness;
    3. Diminished concentration or attention;
    4. Decreased motivation or interest to engage in usual activities;
    5. Insomnia or hypersomnia;
    6. Experience of sleep as unrefreshing or nonrestorative;
    7. Perceived need to struggle to overcome inactivity;
    8. Marked emotional reactivity (e.g., sadness, frustration, or irritability) to feeling fatigued;
    9. Difficulty completing daily tasks attributed to feeling fatigued;
    10. Perceived problems with short-term memory;
    11. Post-exertional malaise lasting several hours.

B. The symptoms cause clinically significant distress or impairment in social, occupational, or other important areas of functioning.

C. There is evidence from the history, physical examination, or laboratory findings that the symptoms are a consequence of cancer or cancer therapy.

D. The symptoms are not primarily a consequence of comorbid psychiatric disorders such as major depression, somatization disorder, somatoform disorder, or delirium.

Reprinted with permission from ONCOLOGY, Melville, NY

cancer patients reported fatigue: 31% a little bit of the time, 23% somewhat of the time, 15% quite a bit of the time, and 8% very much of the time.

To estimate the prevalence of cancer-related fatigue using the proposed diagnostic criteria [1], Cella, Davis, Breitbart, and Curt [11] conducted telephone interviews with a national sample of 379 cancer patients who had received chemotherapy. Seventeen percent of the sample was found to meet formal criteria for cancer-related fatigue (Table 1). This percentage is lower than the previously reported estimates, probably attributable to the methodology used to define fatigue. Previous studies estimated the prevalence of fatigue based on patients who reported any degree of fatigue, regardless of its impact on functioning. In employing diagnostic criteria, Cella et al. [11] required that patients report a significant number of fatigue-related problems and disruption in daily functioning to receive a diagnosis. This helps distinguish the common, everyday fatigue experienced by patients from the more disruptive, debilitating fatigue required to meet formal diagnostic criteria. Clearly, all patients in the latter category would require clinical attention, as would an undetermined portion of those in the former category.

While fatigue is a common experience for cancer patients, it is noteworthy that only 15-25% of patients report diagnosable cancer-related fatigue. Thus, in clinical practice it is important to assess fatigue severity and attempt to differentiate milder from more debilitating fatigue.

Clinical significance

Cancer-related fatigue has been associated with functional limitations and impaired quality of life [2,3,7,8,12]. Women with breast cancer identified fatigue as one of the most distressing cancer-related symptoms [13]. Cella [7] examined a sample of 1025 cancer patients and found that patients reporting high levels of fatigue had very low scores on a quality of life measure. In contrast, patients who did not complain of fatigue had high average scores on the same measure.

Etiology

Fatigue is commonly reported among patients with advanced cancer following chemotherapy or radiotherapy, and among long-term cancer survivors. Fatigue can be one of the first indicators of the presence or recurrence of cancer and tends to increase with the progression of cancer and cancer treatment [14]. Identifying the etiological factors that contribute to fatigue often proves to be complicated, as multiple causes typically coexist. Physiological factors include the direct effects of cancer (e.g. tumor burden), side effects of cancer treatments (e.g., chemotherapy, radiation), secondary conditions (e.g. anemia, malnutrition), and comorbid illnesses. The emotional strain resulting from coping with cancer is also a contributing factor. Depression, apathy, and feelings of hopelessness can also lead to or exacerbate fatigue.

Clinical management

The National Comprehensive Cancer Network (NCCN) has issued Clinical Practice Guidelines for the evaluation and management of fatigue. The authors belong to an NCCN institution and were involved in the development of the Practice Guidelines for Cancer-Related Fatigue (see appendix 1). The following sections on clinical management will review these guidelines, which are being adapted for implementation by the authors at their institution.[1]

The management of cancer-related fatigue requires interdisciplinary evaluation and treatment, given the complex interaction of associated medical, psychological, and social factors that impact fatigue characteristics. Given the

---

[1] Recommendations regarding clinical management set forth by the authors do not necessarily represent views held by NCCN.

prevalence of cancer-related fatigue, routine screening should be conducted with all patients.

Rapid screening

The administration of a brief self-report instrument to screen for the presence and severity of fatigue would facilitate the identification of patients who would benefit from further evaluation and treatment for cancer-related fatigue. An example of a brief screening instrument to identify cancer-related fatigue, pain, emotional distress, and appetite or weight concerns is included in Appendix 2. One or two members of the clinic staff should be designated as being primarily responsible for administering the screening instrument to clinic patients and interpreting patient responses. Patients exceeding predetermined cutoff scores on the screening instrument should be identified by clinic staff for the completion of a more in-depth evaluation by their health care providers. NCCN recommends that patients with moderate or severe fatigue (4 or higher on 0-10 scale) complete a focused history and physical.

Evaluation

The evaluation of cancer patients reporting fatigue should be comprehensive, given the diverse etiological factors and the multidimensional nature of fatigue. Fatigue characteristics, impact on quality of life, and potential physical and psychosocial etiologies should be assessed (NCCN Guidelines). It is recommended that this evaluation include a general component to obtain background information (e.g., demographics, illness characteristics, functional impairments), as well as a fatigue-specific assessment.

Based on the NCCN Practice Guidelines, a comprehensive evaluation should include an assessment of disease status and treatment, as well as an in-depth fatigue assessment (see appendix 3). The fatigue assessment should evaluate fatigue onset, pattern, and duration, change over time, associated or alleviating factors, physical, emotional, and mental symptomatology, and functional interference. Primary factors associated with fatigue should also be assessed, including pain, emotional distress, sleep disturbance, anemia, and hypothyroidism. Patients with primary factors should be evaluated and treated accordingly. Patients with no primary factors should undergo comprehensive assessment.

Comprehensive assessment should include a review of systems, review of medications, assessment of comorbidities, nutritional and metabolic assessment, and an assessment of activity. Specific comorbidities that should be assessed include cardiac, pulmonary, renal, hepatic, and neurological dysfunction and infection. Nutritional and metabolic assessment should evaluate changes in weight and caloric intake, along with fluid electrolyte imbalance. Assessment of activity should examine changes in exercise or activity patterns and deconditioning.

Semi-structured interviews and standardized self-report instruments should be included as part of this evaluation. Several self-report instruments have been developed for the assessment of cancer-related fatigue. The Functional Assessment of Chronic Illness Therapy-Fatigue scale (FACIT-Fatigue) [12] consists of 13 items that measure the impact of fatigue on quality of life. Cella (unpublished data) compared the scores of 2292 cancer patients to those of 1010 individuals from the general population on this scale. These two groups demonstrated two distinct distributions. Cancer patients showed a normal distribution of very low scores, indicating high fatigue ($\underline{M}$ = 23.7 ± 12.6, median = 23.0), while the general population had much less fatigue ($\underline{M}$ = 43.6 ± 9.4, median = 47.0). A discriminant function analysis suggested that an individual with a raw score of 43 and lower (possible raw scores range from 0 to 52) is more likely to be classified as being from the cancer group. The majority of subjects (84.4%) were classified correctly using this cutoff score.

Treatment

Patients who may benefit from intervention to reduce or manage their fatigue should be provided with interdisciplinary treatment. Treatment interventions may vary according to etiologic factors identified.

The NCCN Practice Guidelines for the management of fatigue recommend first treating primary factors associated with fatigue, such as anemia, pain, emotional distress, sleep disturbance, and hypothyroidism. These primary factors should receive clinical attention prior to implementing fatigue management strategies. For example, patients with anemia should receive hematopoietic growth factors when appropriate. Similarly, patients with fatigue secondary to major depression should receive first-line antidepressant therapy, such as an agent in the family of selective serotonin reuptake inhibitors (SSRIs), preferably paired with short-term psychotherapy.

If primary factors are not present or have been addressed, pharmacological, educational, and behavioral interventions have been found to be efficacious in decreasing fatigue [15]. Symptom management strategies, such as activity pacing, exercise, and energy conservation have been used with patients suffering from fatigue that is not amenable to standard treatment interventions.

Based on the NCCN Practice Guidelines, educational interventions and counseling should include information on the known pattern of fatigue during and following cancer treatment, reassurance (when appropriate) that treatment-related fatigue is not an indicator of progression, and fatigue-coping strategies. These strategies include energy conservation techniques, distraction techniques and stress management strategies. Pharmacologic interventions include psychostimulants, antidepressants and steroids. Nonpharmacologic interventions include exercise, restorative therapy, and maintaining good nutrition and sleep hygiene.

Interdisciplinary providers should meet on a weekly basis to review findings from patient evaluations, develop individualized treatment plans, and monitor treatment progress.

Treatment outcome measures

Efficacy of treatment interventions for fatigue can be assessed using patient-based outcome measures. Treatment outcomes can be evaluated on an individual basis and, if patient outcome data can be aggregated, on a clinic basis. The use of standardized questionnaires to assess fatigue to evaluate treatment outcome is recommended. Repeated assessment of outcome measures should be conducted at regular time intervals, ideally prior, during, and following intervention to evaluate treatment efficacy.

Table 2. Standardized instruments for assessment of fatigue

Scale	Domains assessed	Number of items
FACIT-Fatigue Cella, 1997; Yellen et al., 1997	• Symptoms • Functional impact	13
Multidimensional Fatigue Inventory Smets, Garssen, Cull, & de Haes, 1996	• General fatigue • Physical fatigue • Reduced activity • Reduced motivation • Mental fatigue	20
Multidimensional Fatigue Symptom Inventory Stein, Martin, Hann, & Jacobsen, 1998	• Global fatigue • Somatic symptoms • Affective symptoms • Cognitive symptoms • Behavioral symptoms	83
Piper Fatigue Self-Report Scale Piper et al., 1989	• Fatigue severity • Distress • Impact of fatigue	41
Piper Fatigue Self-Report Scale-Short Form Piper et al., 1998	• Behavioral/severity • Affective meaning • Sensory • Cognitive mood	22
Schwartz Cancer Fatigue Scale Schwartz, 1998	• Physical • Emotional • Cognitive • Temporal	28

In selecting measurement tools for the assessment of fatigue, it is important to select instruments that have been examined in terms of reliability and validity with samples of oncology patients. Table 2 lists standardized instruments that assess fatigue and have demonstrated adequate psychometric properties with cancer patients.

Implementing standardized assessment of patients' fatigue can assist with treatment planning, evaluation of treatment interventions, and ultimately with the delivery of better clinical care.

References

1   Cella D, Peterman A, Passik S, Jacobsen P, Breitbart W. Progress toward guidelines for the management of fatigue. Oncology 1998; 12: 369-77

2   Cella D. The Functional Assessment of Cancer Therapy-Anemia (FACT-An) Scale: A new tool for the assessment of outcomes in cancer anemia and fatigue. Semin Hematol 1997; 34S: 13-9

3   Cella D, Tulsky D, Gray G, et al. The functional assessment of cancer therapy scale: Development and validation of the general measure. J Clin Oncol 1993; 11: 570-9

4   Winningham ML, Nail LM, Burke MB, et al. Fatigue and the cancer experience: The state of the knowledge. Oncol Nurs Forum 1994; 21: 23-36

5   Berglund G, Bolund G, Fornander T. Late effects of adjuvant chemotherapy and post-operative radiotherapy on quality of life among breast cancer patients. Eur J Cancer 1991; 27: 1075-81

6   Blesch K, Paice J, Wickham R, et al. Correlates of fatigue in people with breast or lung cancer. Oncol Nurs Forum 1991; 18: 81-7

7   Cella D. Quality of life in cancer patients experiencing fatigue and anemia. Anemia in Oncology 1998; March: 2-4

8   Irvine D, Vincent L, Graydon J, Bubela N, Thompson L. The prevalence and correlates of fatigue in patients receiving treatment with chemotherapy and radiation therapy: A comparison with the fatigue experienced by healthy individuals. Cancer Nurs 1994; 17: 367-78

9   Meyerowitz B, Watkins I, Sparks F. Quality of life for breast cancer patients receiving adjuvant chemotherapy. Am J Nurs 1983; 83: 232-5

10   Vogelzang, NJ, Breitbart W, Cella D, et al. Patient, caregiver, and oncologist perceptions of cancer-related fatigue: results of a tripart assessment survey. The Fatigue Coalition. Semin Hematol 1997; 34S: 4-12

11   Cella D, Davis K, Breitbart W, Curt G. Cancer-related fatigue: Prevalence of proposed diagnostic criteria in a United States sample of cancer survivors. Manuscript under review

12   Yellen S, Cella D, Webster K, Blendowski C, Kaplan E. Measuring fatigue and other anemia-related symptoms with the Functional Assessment of Cancer Therapy (FACT) measurement system. J Pain Symptom Manage 1997; 13: 63-74

13   Longman AJ, Braden CJ, Mishel MH. Side effects burden in women with breast cancer. Cancer Practice 1996; 4: 272-80

14   Greenberg DB. Fatigue. In: Holland J, ed. Psycho-oncology. New York: Oxford University Press 1998; 485-93

15   Portenoy RK, Itri LM. Cancer-related fatigue: Guidelines for evaluation and management. The Oncologist 1999; 4: 1-10

Appendix 1. NCCN Practice Guidelines for Cancer-Related Fatigue

Version 1.2000
18 April 2000

Clinical Trials
NCCN believes the best management of any cancer patient is in a clinical trial. Participation in a clinical trial is especially encouraged.

NCCN Categories of Consensus

Category 1: There is uniform NCCN consensus, based on high-level evidence, that the recommendation is appropriate.

Category 2A: There is uniform NCCN consensus, based on lower-level evidence including clinical experience, that the recommendation is appropriate.

Category 2B: There is nonuniform NCCN consensus (but no major disagreement), based on lower-level evidence including clinical experience, that the recommendation is appropriate.

Category 3: There is major NCCN disagreement that the recommendation is appropriate.

All recommendations are category 2A unless otherwise noted.

The NCCN guidelines are a statement of consensus of its authors regarding their views of currently accepted approaches to treatment. Any clinician seeking to apply or consult any NCCN guideline is expected to use independent medical judgment in the context of individual clinical circumstances to determine any patient's care or treatment. The National Comprehensive Cancer Network makes no warranties of any kind whatsoever regarding their content, use or application and disclaims any responsibility for their application or use in any way.
These guidelines are copyrighted by the National Comprehensive Cancer Network. All rights reserved. These guidelines and the illustrations herein may not be reproduced in any form for any purpose without the express written permission of the NCCN.

Cancer-Related Fatigue   NCCN Practice Guidelines Version 1.2000

DEFINITION OF CANCER-RELATED FATIGUE

Cancer-related fatigue is an unusual, persistent, subjective sense of tiredness related to cancer or cancer treatment that interferes with usual functioning.

STANDARDS OF CARE FOR CANCER-RELATED FATIGUE MANAGEMENT

- Fatigue is a subjective experience that should be actively assessed using patient self-reports and other sources of data.

- Fatigue should be screened, assessed, and managed according to clinical practice guidelines.

- All patients should be screened for fatigue at their initial visit, at regular intervals, and as clinically indicated.

- Fatigue should be recognized, evaluated, monitored, documented, and treated promptly at all stages of disease, during and following treatment.

- Health-care professionals experienced in fatigue evaluation and management should be available for consultation in a timely manner.

- Multidisciplinary institutional committees should be formed to implement guidelines for fatigue management.

- Educational and training programs should be implemented to ensure that health-care professionals have knowledge and skills in the assessment and management of fatigue.

- Patients and families should be informed that management of fatigue is an integral part of total health care.

- Cancer-related fatigue must be included in clinical health outcome studies.

- Quality of fatigue management should be included in institutional continuous quality improvement (CQI) projects.

- Medical care contracts must include reimbursement for the management of fatigue.

Cancer-Related Fatigue

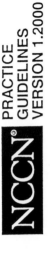

NCCN® PRACTICE GUIDELINES VERSION 1.2000

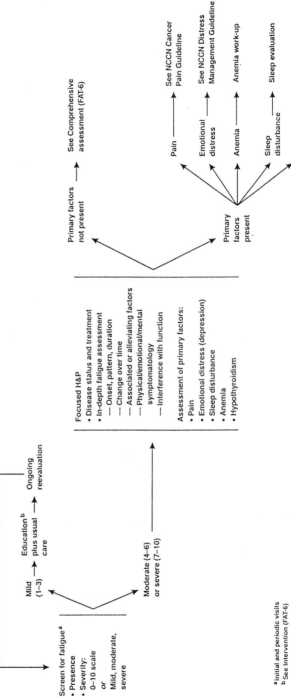

SCREENING

PRIMARY EVALUATION

Screen for fatigue[a]
• Presence
• Severity:
  0–10 scale
  or
  Mild, moderate, severe

Mild (1–3) → Education[b] plus usual care → Ongoing reevaluation

Moderate (4–6) or severe (7–10)

Focused H&P
• Disease status and treatment
• In-depth fatigue assessment
  — Onset, pattern, duration
  — Change over time
  — Associated or alleviating factors
  — Physical/emotional/mental symptomatology
  — Interference with function

Assessment of primary factors:
• Pain
• Emotional distress (depression)
• Sleep disturbance
• Anemia
• Hypothyroidism

Primary factors not present → See Comprehensive assessment (FAT-6)

Primary factors present

Pain → See NCCN Cancer Pain Guideline

Emotional distress → See NCCN Distress Management Guideline

Anemia → Anemia work-up

Sleep disturbance → Sleep evaluation

Hypothyroid → Thyroid evaluation

[a] Initial and periodic visits
[b] See Intervention (FAT-6)

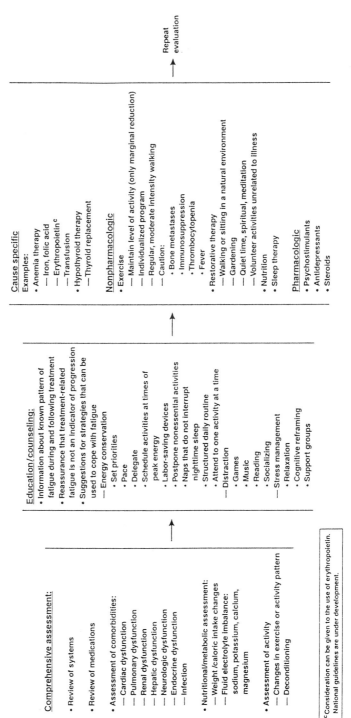

PRIMARY EVALUATION

Comprehensive assessment:

- Review of systems
- Review of medications
- Assessment of comorbidities:
  — Cardiac dysfunction
  — Pulmonary dysfunction
  — Renal dysfunction
  — Hepatic dysfunction
  — Neurologic dysfunction
  — Endocrine dysfunction
  — Infection
- Nutritional/metabolic assessment:
  — Weight/caloric intake changes
  — Fluid electrolyte imbalance:
    sodium, potassium, calcium,
    magnesium
- Assessment of activity
  — Changes in exercise or activity pattern
  — Deconditioning

INTERVENTION

Education/counseling:

- Information about known pattern of
  fatigue during and following treatment
- Reassurance that treatment-related
  fatigue is not an indicator of progression
- Suggestions for strategies that can be
  used to cope with fatigue
  — Energy conservation
    • Set priorities
    • Pace
    • Delegate
    • Schedule activities at times of
      peak energy
    • Labor-saving devices
    • Postpone nonessential activities
    • Naps that do not interrupt
      nighttime sleep
    • Structured daily routine
    • Attend to one activity at a time
  — Distraction
    • Games
    • Music
    • Reading
    • Socializing
  — Stress management
    • Relaxation
    • Cognitive reframing
    • Support groups

Cause specific
Examples:

- Anemia therapy
  — Iron, folic acid
  — Erythropoietin [c]
  — Transfusion
- Hypothyroid therapy
  — Thyroid replacement

Nonpharmacologic

- Exercise
  — Maintain level of activity (only marginal reduction)
  — Individualized program
  — Regular, moderate intensity walking
  — Caution:
    • Bone metastases
    • Immunosuppression
    • Thrombocytopenia
    • Fever
- Restorative therapy
  — Walking or sitting in a natural environment
  — Gardening
  — Quiet time, spiritual, meditation
  — Volunteer activities unrelated to illness
- Nutrition
- Sleep therapy

Pharmacologic

- Psychostimulants
- Antidepressants
- Steroids

Repeat
evaluation

[c] Consideration can be given to the use of erythropoietin.
National guidelines are under development.

Appendix 2. Sample screening instrument

1a. During the past 7 days, how much have you suffered from pain ?

(circle one number)

0   1   2   3   4   5   6   7   8   9   10

Not   Worst I can

at all   imagine

1b. Would you like to speak with someone about this ?   Yes_____   No_____

2a. During the past 7 days, how much have you felt tired, fatigued, or "washed out"?

(circle one number)

0   1   2   3   4   5   6   7   8   9   10

Not   Worst I can

at all   imagine

2b. Would you like to speak with someone about this ?   Yes_____   No_____

3a. During the past 7 days, how much have you felt depressed or distressed ?

(circle one number)

0   1   2   3   4   5   6   7   8   9   10

Not   Worst I can

at all   imagine

3b. Would you like to speak with someone about this ?   Yes_____   No_____

4a. During the past 7 days, how concerned have you been about your appetite or weight ?

(circle one number)

0   1   2   3   4   5   6   7   8   9   10

Not   Worst I can

at all   imagine

4b. Would you like to speak with someone about this ?   Yes_____   No_____

Appendix 3. Sample interview for fatigue-specific assessment

On average, how often do you feel tired, fatigued, or "washed out"? _____
      Rate from 0 (not at all) to 10 (all of the time)

On average, how severe is your fatigue? _____
      Rate from 0 (no fatigue) to 10 (very severe)

How severe is your fatigue at its worst? _____
      Rate from 0 (no fatigue) to 10 (very severe)

How severe is your fatigue at its least? _____
      Rate from 0 (no fatigue) to 10 (very severe)

Is your fatigue pretty constant or does it seem to come and go? _____

When did you first notice fatigue? _____ (date)
      Before or after cancer diagnosis? _____
      Before or after cancer treatments? _____

Did your fatigue seem to begin suddenly or more gradually? _____

Does your fatigue seem worse in the morning, afternoon, or evening? _____

When do you have the most energy? _____

What do you think is causing your fatigue? _____

What helps to reduce your fatigue? _____

    If no factors identified:

        Sleep? _____
        Exercise? _____
        Relaxation? _____
        Cutting back on activities? _____

What have you tried to improve your energy? _____

    Has anything worked? _____

What makes your fatigue worse? _____

    If no factors identified:

        Stress? _____
        Trying to do too much? _____

Which of the following feelings or problems have you noticed?

Physical symptoms		Emotional symptoms		Cognitive symptoms	
Worn-out		Overwhelmed		Hard to concentrate	
No energy		Sad		Hard to think clearly	
Exhausted		Listless		Hard to remember things	
Weakness		Frustrated		Hard to pay attention	
Sleepiness		Helpless		Cloudy thinking	

What activities does your fatigue interfere with?

_____

How do family members/friends respond to your fatigue?

_____

Have you talked with your health-care providers about your fatigue?

_____

    Were they helpful? _____

Subject Index